Staying Healthy in the *Fast Lane*

9 Simple Steps to Optimal Health
and Real Healthcare Reform

Kirk Hamilton

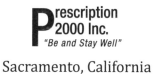

Prescription
2000 Inc.
"Be and Stay Well"

Sacramento, California

Prescription 2000, Inc.
3301 Alta Arden, Suite 3
Sacramento, CA 95825

Visit our Web site at www.Prescription2000.com

Printed in the United States of America

First Edition: July 2011

10 9 8 7 6 5 4 3 2 1

Library of Congress Control Number: 2011902260

ISBN 978-1-890302-11-5

Cover design by Jamie O'Neal with modifications
by Konstantin Koryaka and Gwyn Snider
Interior Book Design by Integrative Ink
with modifications by GKS Creative

What Others Say About Kirk Hamilton's
Staying Healthy in the *Fast Lane*

"The time has come for every American to take charge of their health destiny and give up the false notion that doctors and drugs will save us as we commit slow suicide with food. The reliance on drugs is a proven failure and we have an overweight, sickly, and cancer-prone population to prove it. Kirk Hamilton does his homework; *Staying Healthy in the Fast Lane* by Kirk will put you on track to a long, healthy life."

Joel Fuhrman, MD
Best-selling author of *Eat To Live*
Family Physician and Nutritional Researcher
DrFuhrman.com

"Kirk Hamilton has developed an objective, precise, and clearly defined protocol for not only staying healthy but also optimizing your physical, emotional, and psychological health. There are no shortcuts, but once you begin to accept and implement his simple suggestions, you'll be on the path for a lifetime of renewed health. A very powerful book, and one that I've added to my health library."

Dave Scott
Six-time Ironman Triathlon Champion
Dave Scott, Inc. Boulder, Colorado

"Kirk Hamilton has an excellent reputation in integrative medicine and in addition is an intelligent medical reporter and writer. He uses many years of clinical experience in writing this new book. It is an excellent source of information for the patient and clinician alike. In addition, the book provides easy to understand guidelines for staying healthy in the modern world. I recommend that you read and use this helpful information."

Burton M. Berkson, MD, MS, PhD
The Integrative Medical Center of New Mexico
Author of *The Lipoic Acid Breakthrough*

"This book contains an important and often overlooked perspective on the diseases of civilization. More importantly, it offers a detailed and practical method for enhancing and maintaining health that would be appropriate for people of all ages."

Robert Krikorian, PhD
Associate Professor of Psychiatry & Behavioral Neuroscience
Director of the Cognitive Disorders Center
University of Cincinnati

"I love the simplicity with which Kirk has addressed the health problems we face at the societal and individual levels and also the remedy to rectify them. The strategy is basic, straightforward, entirely effective, backed up by thousands of scientific articles in the literature on the importance of a whole-food, plant-based diet, a consistent and progressive exercise routine, and an overall positive approach to life. Anyone who is afflicted with chronic disease or who wants to avoid such calamities in the first place should read and apply Kirk's methods."

John E. Lewis, PhD
Assistant Professor
Director of Research for Complementary and Integrative Medicine
Associate Director, Medical Wellness Center,
University of Miami School of Medicine

"Kirk has an eternal spring of healthy information unlike anyone I know. He is passionate and brilliant and 100% committed to helping YOU reach your optimum health. Read and enjoy this book!"

Rip Esselstyn
Texas Fireman
Former World Class Professional Triathlete
Author of *Engine 2 Diet*

"Information overload is wearing us all down. Health-wise, how can we figure out what really matters and what really works? Kirk Hamilton's book provides the answers. Everyone should read it and apply its wisdom to their lives."

Mark Scholz, MD
Medical Director, Prostate Oncology Specialists
Marina Del Rey, California
Co-author of *Invasion of the Prostate Snatchers*

"As we get older, life passes by with increasing velocity. Thank goodness Kirk Hamilton has condensed the important elements of staying healthy so we really can fit it into our busy lives. His advice is practical and doable—so just do it and stay healthy."

Peter Starr
Film Producer
Chairman, *Healing Arts Education Foundation*

"Kirk Hamilton has synthesized the best scientific health information with his extensive knowledge as a medical clinician and healer. His health manual is a prescription for getting well and staying well, replete with practical 'steps' that any person can take to start the process of recovering their mind and body. Read the book now and get started on your road to recovery!"

Martin P. Gallagher, MD, DC
Board Certified Family Physician
Physician Acupuncturist
Medical Wellness Associates

"Don't look to the White House or the Senate for healthcare reform. Turn instead to Kirk Hamilton's comprehensive guide *Staying Healthy in the Fast Lane*. It's a real page-turner that explains with clarity, detail, and passion how we can (and must) take responsibility for our own healthcare reform. The steps that Hamilton outlines for us are medically sound and well worth taking."

R. Keith McCormick, DC
U.S. Olympic Team member
Ironman Triathlon competitor
Author of *The Whole-Body Approach to Osteoporosis*

"Kirk has brought together science with real-life experiences. His ability to bring in his personal life adds a touch to this book that others do not have, yet allows the readers to relate to circumstances they may be going through themselves."

Stella L. Volpe, PhD, RD, LD/N, FACSM
Professor and Chair
Drexel University Department of Nutrition

"Thank you for this well-thought-out book targeted to help the confused and overwhelmed typical American patient. The clearly defined steps you describe will take many people by the hand and lead them to good health and well-being. This book will be a must-read for patients in our clinic."

Jeanne Drisko, MD, CNS, FACN
Riordan Endowed Professor of Orthomolecular Medicine
Director, Program in Integrative Medicine
Complementary and Alternative Therapies
University of Kansas Medical Center

"The goal of most of my customers in the fitness industry over the past 30 years has been to lose and maintain weight, exercise to health, and alleviate stress while conducting a busy life with severe time constraints. Kirk Hamilton has provided a concise, compact prescription with a template for just that population. We can use his book as the blueprint in the fitness industry to educate and assist busy people to the results and lifestyle they desire. Kirk is a dedicated researcher and medical practitioner who brings the best of research, medical, and alternative information, matched with his passion and intensity. This book is an excellent summary for the lay public and fitness professional. For those looking to simplify the plethora of information available on health, weight loss, and exercise, Kirk's book is a quick recipe to success."

Galen Miler, President
Millennium Sport Clubs

"I have known Kirk Hamilton for several years. Kirk has supported family, friends, and strangers alike in venues in and out of the health field. He is a man of his word. After reading *Staying Healthy in the Fast Lane*, I realized immediately the value given in his TRIAD Wellness Program's 9

Simple Steps to Optimal Health. If you care about your future health or the health of a loved one, this book is a must-read."

Michael J. Papa, President of Breit International, Inc.
Author of *Good Communication: A Lost Art*

"Kirk Hamilton has been someone that I have respected and turned to for knowledge over the past 15 years. His latest book *Staying Healthy in the Fast Lane* is another example of his invaluable approach to health and well-being. What is so often neglected in a health program is the individual's responsibility to make healthy choices. So many people are looking for the magic combination of supplements that will undo all of the harm that their lifestyle habits cause. Kirk's latest publication gives the reader all of the information that they need, but also emphasizes that the first line of defense against chronic disease is choosing a healthy lifestyle and diet. This is a must read for anyone looking to improve their health using a common sense approach well steeped in science."

Emmett J. Hughes, DC, MS
Associate Professor of Basic Science
University of Bridgeport College of Chiropractic

"*Staying Healthy in the Fast Lane* is solid and exciting information to help us all stay in good health. Kirk Hamilton searches for answers with untiring zeal. It is to the advantage of pharmaceutical companies to turn 'symptoms,' that can be corrected by diet, into diseases that are then treated with drugs. By following Kirk's guidelines, you can escape the trap and have a vibrantly healthy life. Kirk is a searcher, researcher, and a teacher of good health in an untiring, exciting way. This is a wonderful book that will help thousands of people have a happier, healthier life. Read it and follow it—you will be glad you did."

Barbara Stitt, PhD
Author of *Food and Behavior*

"The landscape of health is changing, with a comprehensive integrative approach to healthcare emerging. Staying Healthy in the Fast Lane is a valuable resource for today's families, as it informs and inspires with smart, sensible and savvy tips to help protect and restore the health of our loved ones."

Robyn O'Brien, Author of *The Unhealthy Truth*
Founder, AllergyKids Foundation

Staying Healthy in the *Fast Lane*

9 Simple Steps to Optimal Health
and Real Healthcare Reform

To my beloved mother, Adela, for her "you can do it!" belief in me.
I know you are with me every day...

To my beautiful daughter Mya, Ken and
their children, Ava Jane and Drury,
you inspire G-Paw to keep working at his dream
of making this a better and healthier world.

Contents

9 Simple Steps to Optimal Health

TRIAD Wellness Program

3 Phases x 3 Steps

I. TRIAD Diet Program:

1. **EAT whole, unprocessed foods** (90 percent or more as plant foods, if not all plant foods).
2. **EAT** at least half your food intake as **vegetables**.
3. **ELIMINATE** all **dairy products** or eat from the **Basic Elimination Diet (BED)** for at least one month.

II. TRIAD Exercise Program:

4. **DO** a half-hour minimum of daily **aerobic exercise**.
5. **DO strength training** (circuit training) fifteen to thirty minutes, three to four days per week.
6. **DO flexibility training** (tai chi, yoga, Pilates, stretching) ten to sixty minutes daily.

III. TRIAD Mind-Body:

7. **BE thankful** for five minutes, morning and evening.
8. **SIT quietly** for fifteen to sixty minutes daily.
9. **IMAGINE your ideal health** and life daily for five to fifteen minutes. Think about what you want, not about what you don't want. Write it down. Picture it!

It is an honor to have Dr. David Jenkins write the Foreword to this book. I have been fortunate enough not only to have read his scientific work but also to have interviewed him on multiple occasions over the last fifteen years. His credentials and responsibilities speak for themselves—among them: Canada Research Chair in Nutrition and Metabolism; Professor of Medicine and Nutritional Sciences, University of Toronto; Director, Risk Factor Modification Center, St. Michael's Hospital, Toronto, Canada; and the developer of the Glycemic Index and Dietary Portfolio. That said, what I am most impressed with, and inspired by, is his commitment to preventing and reversing chronic disease with a lifestyle approach that protects the environment and other life forms, utilizing scientific plant-based nutrition. His thoughtful leadership in this arena will help preserve mankind's health and our mutual home, planet Earth, for generations to come.

—Kirk Hamilton

Foreword

In 1988, Boyd Eaton published "Stone Agers in the Fast Lane." It was a call to return to a Paleolithic diet much higher in meat and animal products than eaten in the 1980s or even today. Now Kirk Hamilton has written *Staying Healthy in the Fast Lane,* a call to limit the dependence of Homo sapiens on animal foods.

Both publications share a common theme: that the modern lifestyle is not in keeping with the requirements of human physiology. The evidence for this mismatch comes from the figures for obesity and diabetes now in evidence in Western nations, with diabetes alone at 8 to 9 percent in North America and predicted to double in the next twenty years. If this scenario holds true, we will see an increase in renal failure, blindness, and cardiovascular disease together with many cancers. For these reasons, public awareness must be stimulated, and much research undertaken, with translation of this knowledge to the public so that effective preventive strategies are put in place.

Kirk's focus has been to stem those lifestyle and dietary factors, which he sees as the problem in both industrialized and developing countries:

- Increased consumption of animals products
- Increased consumption of added fats and oils
- Increased consumption of added calorie sweeteners
- An *increase* in processed grains worldwide, with a *decrease* in developing countries of the percentage of calories from grains compared to other food calories
- A decrease in physical activity

The first diet rule in Kirk's *9 Simple Steps to Optimal Health* is for 90 percent or more of the diet to be unprocessed whole plant foods. The other 10 percent is optional as animal foods, but it is not necessary and not recommended as such.

Kirk is clearly committed to plant-based nutrition as a major theme of the book—not only for chronic disease prevention and reversal but also for protection of the ecology of the planet for a world population approaching 7 billion people.

This aspect of the book is, for me, of major importance. It is also what differentiates this book from other good health manuals. We are losing possibly one species every fifteen minutes. By 2050, the rainforest will be destroyed and all fish stocks will be depleted. Mankind must change his ways not only for himself but also for his planet. This book shows that by eating in a way that protects other life forms and the environment, we can maximize our health and also prevent and reverse the epidemic of modern day chronic disease.

David J.A. Jenkins, MD, PhD, DSc

Preface

This book *really* started in the last quarter of my physician assistant training at U.C. Davis in 1983. One of our projects was to outline a book. I remember vaguely calling it *Lifestyling*. The concept of the book was about prevention of disease and staying well by having a good diet, exercising, and doing some stress reduction.

Throughout my more than quarter-century of being a practicing PA (physician assistant), I have always been a nutrition research junkie. I have also written newsletters, given talks, done some radio, and have tried to practice what I preached by living a lifestyle that involves a lot of exercise, a pretty good diet, and reasonable attempts at stress reduction...well, two out of three isn't too bad! Actually, I feel so blessed to have followed this path. If I hadn't been working on those three key aspects of wellness all these years, I probably would have been in a whole lot of trouble health-wise by now, especially because of how much pressure and work I put on myself.

Within six months of working in my first "alternative medicine" practice in 1983, I came up with a one-page handout for patients called *Optimal Health*. There were six key components: (1) Spirituality, (2) Exercise, (3) Nutrition, (4) Stress, (5) Environment, and (6) Self-Care. This handout summarized what I thought an individual had to practice daily in order to be in "optimal health." I have it on my wall today in my home office. I still believe in 90–95 percent of the recommendations more than a quarter of a century later. They are really the fundamental principles in *Staying Healthy in the Fast Lane*.

In the mid-1980s, while still practicing as a PA in a nutrition prevention-oriented primary care medical practice in Sacramento, I also became a massage therapist. During those two to three years of training, I received an overview of Chinese medicine as well as firsthand experience of how powerful our emotions are in affecting our health. It was clearly evident that if emotions were not expressed appropriately, they could cause disease. During this same time, I attempted to start an early version of a health coaching business called Lifestyling. I wasn't successful, but always at my core, I realized real healing and wellness occurred *outside* the exam room. It was extremely clear that what people do daily in the three areas of diet, exercise, and stress management, or the mind/ body connection, are the keys to health and wellness.

It had dawned on me by then that most of the patients I and most other health professionals saw really would not need to be seen if they effectively implemented good diet, exercise, and mind-body practices. Little did I know then that those three components—diet, exercise, and stress management—would turn into the **TRIAD Wellness Program** and the *9 Simple Steps to Optimal Health* more than two decades later, and are the foundations for achieving the goal of this book...for you to be well and stay that way in the busy, modern world and use health professionals and related services minimally.

I have always had this book in my consciousness but felt a greater, more immediate passion between 1989 and 2004 to educate health professionals on current nutrition and prevention research. Why? Because working in an alternative or integrative medicine practice we were always criticized for not practicing scientific medicine. So for those fifteen years, I reviewed one to two hundred medical journal papers each month, summarized the research into newsletters, books, and databases, and did more than 650 interviews of medical researchers from all over the world on current medical research in nutrition and prevention. I learned a lot, earned a good reputation among my peers, worked very hard, and sold that business (Clinical Pearls) in 2004.

Very thankfully, that research, found in the "Clinical Pearls" database, is alive and well thanks to Raj Chopra Sr. of Tishcon Corporation. Not only has Tishcon Corporation kept the database going, but they also made it better and free to health professionals and the public at Vitasearch.com. I continued to do "Expert Interviews" for Vitasearch and am approaching one thousand interviews since 1994, when I started. All that data and experiences regarding nutrition and prevention research are intertwined in this book, *Staying Healthy in the Fast Lane*.

Over the next four years (2004–2008), I continued to see patients and conduct written "Expert Interviews" for Vitasearch.com. During this same time period, my mother developed pulmonary fibrosis. Like so many sons and daughters nowadays, my siblings and I took care of our mother. Our goal was to assist her in remaining as independent as possible, with the least amount of invasive medical intervention, and to keep her at home, surrounded by her loved ones, at the time of her passing. We did it. And we did a good job. I learned a lot firsthand about what I had been seeing in my patients for the last ten years or so: not only chronic health problems in my patients but also a new problem of how children and spouses now have to take care of an ever-growing unhealthy, aging population with a multitude of chronic diseases.

These patient care experiences, along with taking care of my mother, had a profound impact on me. These experiences reinforced the need in my own life as I passed the half-century mark, as well as in my patients (and society), that the daily practice of these three lifestyle components (diet, exercise, and stress management) were not only very important for staying well but also for our society to remain viable socially and economically as it rapidly ages.

During those four years, a *burn* deep inside me was starting to develop again. It had a sense of urgency and renewed passion to it—to really get back into the health education game and make the impact that I believed was possible. But this time my focus was on the public first and professionals second. The time was now for a book for everyone—not just health professionals interested in nutrition and prevention research but for people like my patients. As I mentioned previously, it was becoming even more obvious to me that most of my patients really wouldn't need to be in my office and the offices of others if they practiced some daily basic health promoting principles. In fact, it has become obvious to me that the whole *healthcare reform debate* has nothing to do with the government really. *It has to do with you and me practicing these basic principles of wellness on a daily basis.* **Healthcare reform is your personal responsibility**. That is a major theme in this book.

When my mother passed, which was the most beautiful family experience of my life, it became very clear that it was time for me to embark on this book that I have had in my consciousness, practiced personally, researched, and taught about since 1983. By the end of 2008, it was "go time." The only thing standing in my way to writing this book was my own fear of failure and more hard work.

Then things began to fall into place. The universe started sending the opportunities my way. The pieces for this book came together quickly. I designed a five-part *Staying Healthy* lecture series (*Staying Healthy in the Fast Lane, Reversing Diabetes, Reversing Obesity, Reversing Heart Disease, and Healthy Aging*) and began to teach again. It reminded me how much I loved and missed being up in front of people, sharing solid self-help information. It also reminded me of how life-giving and healing teaching and sharing information with others is for me.

The ultimate goal in this *Staying Healthy* series was to show where the modern, industrialized world was heading with the ever-increasing incidence of chronic diseases and their human and economic costs. My intent for these seminars was to show that lifestyle factors, especially dietary changes, that have occurred over the last fifty to one hundred years as the world industrialized, are the main causes of these largely preventable chronic diseases (heart disease, diabetes, obesity, etc.), *not bad genes*. From researching, preparing, and refining this five-part series, along with interviewing wonderful physicians, researchers, and book authors (*Staying Healthy Today Show*), it became evident that not only were these chronic diseases preventable, but many were also reversible through aggressive lifestyle practices.

Now, after hundreds of hours of not only writing and editing, but more research, multiple rewrites, and the hardest part, cutting down a wordy, disjointed 450-page manuscript in half, the book you are reading is the end result.

There is one additional and important aspect to the development of this book that is worth mentioning. In a way, this is a type of autobiography about me: your basic middle-aged male who is right in the middle of that time when men get chronic diseases and are also very busy with a lot of self-inflicted pressure and self-worth issues—a prescription for health problems.

In hindsight, there are several reasons why I didn't start writing this book twenty-five years ago. But one became evident after I had received my first unsolicited AARP mailing as I approached fifty (now fifty-four). The reason the timing wasn't right to create this book in my twenties or thirties was that I personally needed to be practicing these *Staying Healthy* principles for several decades in order to see and feel clearly their effects on my own life before sharing them confidently and passionately with the world.

It has become abundantly clear to me, all the scientific research aside, that living my very physically active lifestyle with a whole-food, plant-strong diet, along with my acceptable but not great attempts at stress reduction, are paying off. I firmly believe that had I not been led to nutrition and preventive medicine as a profession and had not lived this lifestyle, I would be in serious trouble with my health right now. That is why I know to the core of my being that the information in this book really works.

The timing for me to write this book is perfect—for my own life, because of my experiences and where the world is now with the epidemic of chronic disease, rapid industrialization, and the expanding aging population.

I promise you that if you work at these *Staying Healthy* principles consistently, good things will happen to enhance your vitality, slow your aging process, and reduce your risk of chronic disease.

Acknowledgments

I am in deep gratitude to my family, especially my daughter, Mya; my three siblings, Jock, Denise, and Theresa; and my aunt Amber, for understanding my "absence" as I have pursued this vision.

To my co-workers at Health Associates Medical Group of more than twenty-five years for putting up with my restlessness, changing schedules, and moods as I followed my dream—especially my boss, friend, and supervising physician, Michael J. Kwiker, DO.

To all the wonderful clinicians and researchers who have inspired me, taught me, and given me creative ideas on the big picture of nutritional and preventive medicine, especially Jeffrey Bland, PhD; Alan Gaby, MD; and Jonathan Wright, MD.

To Raj Chopra Sr. of Tishcon Corporation for keeping *Clinical Pearls* and the *Expert Interviews* alive, as they are a great service and a significant part of my life's work.

To Galen Miler, Gerardo Perez, and Michael Desmond, my closest friends, business confidants, and most importantly people who really believed in me when I was struggling to believe in myself.

To my former wife and close friend, Karen Rae Hamilton, who put up with the *Clinical Pearls* years, and to this day is one of my greatest supporters.

To Lynn Boro, my dear friend and spiritual adviser, for guiding me along my path of self-fulfillment.

To the editors of this book, Courtney Arnold, Jodi Brandon, Renee Johnson, and Stephanee Killen. Taking my information-dense, over-detailed writing and putting it into a comprehensible format that a real person could read is a significant accomplishment and very much appreciated.

To Stephanee Killen, senior editor and designer at *Integrative Ink*, for guiding me step by step through the last phases of putting this book together.

To Gwyn Snider of GKS Creative for getting this book print-ready.

To Mark Pitzele of Book Printing Revolution for providing me the last minute resources to complete this book.

To Konstantin Koryaka for last minute graphics and formatting changes.

I want to thank the following current book authors, clinicians, and researchers who have created a vision for a practical and viable healthcare model that can not only *slow and prevent chronic disease but also actually reverse it,* while at the same time preserving the ecology of the planet as a whole. James W. Anderson, MD; Neal D. Barnard, MD; Dan Buettner; T. Colin Campbell, PhD; Caldwell B. Esselstyn Jr., MD; Rip Esselstyn; Richard M. Fleming, MD; Joel Fuhrman, MD; David J.A. Jenkins, MD, PhD, DSc; Daphne Miller, MD; Dean Ornish, MD; John Robbins; Paul and Barbara Stitt; Makoto Suzuki, MD; Bradley J. Willcox, MD; and D. Craig Willcox, PhD.

To Hodan Farah Wells, PhD, and Jean Buzby, PhD, from the USDA's Economic Research Service for helping me with the graphs showing the U.S. dietary consumption patterns over the last century.

To Dr. David J.A. Jenkins for taking time out of his very busy schedule to write the Foreword for this book.

Lastly, and most importantly, I am so deeply grateful to you, Mom and Dad, for inspiring me to try and do good, work hard, and never give up. I wish you were here...and you are!

Introduction

When I am in a grocery store and see a stressed-out parent dragging an overweight or obese child with one hand and pushing a shopping cart full of empty-calorie, sweet-fat foods with the other, I feel deeply saddened. When I flip on the television to watch the Olympic Games, symbol of humankind's greatest physical potential, and see commercials advertising high-calorie fast food from major U.S. corporations, I shake my head. And when I look at a group of overweight adults, and now children, and recognize the obvious risk factors for vascular disease, diabetes, and other *dangerous yet avoidable* chronic diseases, I am motivated to make a difference.

Being an expert in any field means that sometimes you see things the average person cannot. In my case, I need only look at a person's outward physical state and observe the things they are doing in order to predict what degenerative diseases they have or will eventually develop. I am a physician assistant who has been practicing primary care, nutrition, and integrative medicine since 1983. I know that lifestyle habits and actions have a one-to-one correlation with how we look and feel and what diseases we get.

Sometimes, when I see how much people are suffering physically, mentally, and emotionally from unnecessary illness, I want to just grab them and say, "This doesn't have to happen! You can change this! It is easier than you think! These common diseases are not inevitable!"

I want to show them the evidence that the degenerative diseases we, as a culture, have come to accept as part of the aging process do not have to exist to anywhere near the degree that they do in today's modern society. Or better yet, have them read about the lifestyle habits of successfully aging populations from around the world who are living functional and meaningful lives into their eighties, nineties, and one hundreds with minimal chronic disease. For those of you who say, "It's their lucky genes!"—no, it's not! Their children, grandchildren, and relatives who adopt the modern, Western lifestyle get these chronic diseases as soon as they start living this lifestyle, either by immigrating to the West or as the Western lifestyle comes to them due to globalization. Same genes, different lifestyle—opposite and devastating results!

We all have the power to create health and wellness right now. The best part about all of this is that it isn't even difficult—at least not the know-how. The major chronic diseases of developed countries (heart disease; diabetes; stroke; bone loss; arthritis; aging eye disorders such as macular degeneration, glaucoma, and cataracts; aging neurological disorders such as Alzheimer's and Parkinson's; and most cancers) are largely preventable, are sometimes reversible, or can, at the very least, be significantly delayed or diminished in severity by practicing what I call the *9 Simple Steps to Optimal Health.* It is that simple! I will show you these nine simple steps that are guaranteed to improve your health if you apply them daily and consistently!

My Challenge to You

I am going to challenge you on every page in this book to take the healthcare reform debate out of the hands of the politicians and take charge of creating your own healthcare insurance or security. If we all practiced these *9 Simple Steps to Optimal Health* we could save billions of dollars as a country, be so much more productive work-wise, and be more present to our families and loved ones. Collectively we could focus our energies and talents on solving the world's difficult problems. The first step is to educate yourself with understandable, credible, and practical health information. That is my commitment to you: to provide health information that is non-hyped, factual, and usable in the *busy, modern world.* The second step is to stop blaming others for your present health situation. Stop blaming big pharmaceutical companies, the fast- and processed-food industries, health insurance companies, your employer, corporate agribusiness, the "hospital-industrial complex," and, yes, good old Uncle Sam. The third step is to take daily action and practice these health principles consistently and with intention.

Personal Responsibility: The Key to Being Healthy

Yes, government officials could obviously be less wasteful, more efficient and accountable, and not give subsidies to make unhealthy food cheaper, and on and on. But the truth is you can take the issue out of their hands *immediately* by living these simple lifestyle practices right *now!* The last time I ate a meal, Uncle Sam didn't grab my fork and stick it in a fat, juicy steak or grab a piece of pizza and stuff it into my mouth. The last time I turned on the TV, Uncle Sam didn't chain me to my couch so I couldn't use the exercycle or treadmill during my favorite show. Uncle Sam didn't make me take the escalator versus the steps or park as close as possible when I go shopping so that I would not have to walk farther... *Are you catching my drift?* You are in charge of all of that! Quit blaming the government—or anyone else—for your health! Make simple, good choices about what you put into your mouth every time you eat and commit to moving every day, and our current healthcare crisis will become a non-issue. We will become more productive as a nation, and you will have more time and money to be you. Those industries that don't have our real health interests at heart will have no power. If we stay well, insurance companies, big pharma, and factory medicine have no muscle. If daily, we make the right whole-food choices and exercise, not only do we stay healthy, but agribusiness and the fast-food industries will then have to change or die. It could happen literally overnight with the simple daily choices we make to feed ourselves.

The onus is on you once you educate yourself and understand some basic principles. Once you are knowledgeable, you are the conductor of your healthcare journey. Once you understand and really believe that there are cultures and individuals who have minimal chronic disease, you will begin to see the fundamental lifestyle practices that allow them to achieve this state of health. Once you understand, by simply looking at the figures in this book, how the modern diet and lifestyle have changed over the last fifty to one hundred years, setting the stage for these diseases, then the practicing of these *9 Simple Steps to Optimal Health* is a "no-brainer."

Disease Care vs. Preventive Care

You might ask, "If it is so obvious, Kirk, why isn't everybody already doing these things and experiencing health and vitality even into old age?" There are several reasons, but one main reason is that *our healthcare model is focused on disease treatment, not on prevention.* This is a backward model that can only lead to more chronic disease, more suffering, and more unnecessary medical expenditures. We financially reward people to let disease happen and then treat it. We don't compensate people and professionals for preventing these chronic diseases in the first place. We don't give economic incentives for patients to stay well or to businesses to keep their employees well. Insurance companies have no incentive to encourage prevention of disease if they keep raising premiums to treat more chronic diseases and we (individuals, businesses, and government) keep paying the premiums. So with our current healthcare model, unless the "pain" is great enough or the country goes bankrupt, it can't and won't lead to necessary change.

I must say, though, that as a society, we may be approaching the pain threshold that will make us act. My hope is that your "pain" and openness to learn will lead you to look at, try to understand, and most importantly begin practicing these *9 Simple Steps to Optimal Health*, or what I call the **TRIAD Wellness Program**.

Who Is This Book For?

When I began to write this book, I imagined that I would be talking to you, the individual reader, as I would one of my patients.

At the beginning, I figured that I would just put the final sections of this book down on paper in the shortest, most succinct manner possible so that you could get started right away applying these simple principles to achieve immediate results. I still very much want that for you. Yet for many people, a deeper understanding is important because it puts a reason behind the recommendations.

Many people jump on and off healthful practices because they don't really understand how health works; they are very frustrated and looking for a "quick fix" that never really works in the long run. I strongly believe that if you understand why we are unhealthy as individuals, a country, and now the world, and understand the "how to" of these *9 Simple Steps to Optimal Health*, you will be able to stay on a positive, health-promoting lifestyle. The truth is that good health is much simpler than investing in the stock market, running a business, or being a working mother with three children. Good health is simple, not rocket science. You will experience an immediate return if you just keep practicing these principles 80 to 90 percent of the time.

Citizenship and Health: What's the Connection?

To me it is important for each American to take care of his or her own health. If we as a country followed the **TRIAD Wellness** approach using the *9 Simple Steps to Optimal Health*, it would save our country billions of dollars and greatly enhance worksite productivity, helping our economy and increasing our ability to compete in the global marketplace. Having a healthy workforce and a strong economy can only enhance our security as a nation. Good health is a goal each American should have. *Being healthy is being patriotic.*

Leading the World to Good Health

With this example of positively changing the health of the United States, and thereby improving our economy, work productivity, quality of life, and environment, we (the United States) can be the world leader we should be. In this free market system full of positive, health-promoting entrepreneurship, in conjunction with "lean" government, we can show other countries how to help their own people be healthy and productive and reduce this needless toll of suffering and cost that comes from chronic diseases related to the modern lifestyle. The message in this book is not just meant for the individual or even for my own country; it is meant for the whole world.

Staying Healthy in the *Fast Lane*: "You Can Do It!"

My mother was a wonderful and inspiring woman. Even in the days before she passed, she never lost her positive spirit or her will to succeed. One of my favorite memories of her is huffing and puffing, attached to her oxygen tubing and using her walker as she slowly crossed my dance floor, cheering herself on. "You can do it, Del," she would say. "You can do it!"

My message to you is that "**You can do it**!" The time is *now* to change the way we practice medicine and the way we maintain our own health. The nutrition and exercise data are there; the examples of successfully aging cultures living with minimal chronic disease are there. All that is left is for us to just do it! I know you can! Come join me!

Part I:

The Problem

Chapter 1

URBANIZATION, THE MODERN LIFESTYLE, AND CHRONIC DISEASE

What's the Problem?

Chronic diseases, such as heart disease, cancer, diabetes, high blood pressure, stroke, arthritis, bone loss, and degenerative neurologic and ocular diseases are increasing worldwide as the world urbanizes. These chronic conditions account for 70 percent of all deaths in the United States and 60 percent of all deaths worldwide.[1] In the Unites States, 75 percent of the healthcare budget is used to treat chronic diseases.[2] These diseases result in enormous healthcare costs, loss of work productivity, and human suffering. These chronic conditions can be significantly reduced, their progression slowed, and some virtually eliminated by lifestyle changes involving diet, increased physical activity, and positive mental conditioning. Pharmaceutical approaches can only treat symptoms but do not correct the underlying causes of these conditions. In addition, adverse drugs reactions (ADRs) are among the top-ten leading causes of death in the United States.[3]

Why so Much Chronic Disease?

As countries urbanize (move from an agrarian lifestyle to cities) and as manufacturing, transportation, and marketing improve, more processed foods, which are high in caloric density and low in nutrient density, are consumed. This is why the world has seen an increase in "empty" calorie consumption, even in countries where food shortages exist. Also, individuals in urban areas are generally less physically active and have a more chronically stressful lifestyle.

Individual calorie availability has increased between four and five hundred calories per day in the United States over the last century.[4] Between 1970 and 2008, calorie intake has increased from 2,168 to 2,673 calories per day (a 505-calorie increase).[5]

It takes 3,500 calories to equal a pound. Therefore, we have been consuming almost a pound extra in calories per week over the last forty years. This is why the United States has an epidemic of overweight issues and associated diseases.

The major reasons for this calorie increase in the United States come from **five major dietary changes and patterns over the last century** (see illustrations at end of chapter 1):

1. A continued increase in total **meat** consumption, with red meat consumption decreasing and poultry consumption increasing.[6]
2. A dramatic increase in added **fats and oils** to foodstuffs.[7]
3. A continued, steady increase in **calorie sweeteners**, more so from corn sweeteners now than the cane and beet sugars of the past.[8]
4. A dramatic increase in **cheese** consumption.[9]
5. An increase in **grains** since the early 1970s, of which 85 percent are **refined grains**, with "sweet-fat" calories added. (Note: Though grain consumption is higher today than the 1970s, total grain consumption in the early 1900s was greater than it is today, with four to five hundred fewer total calories per day consumed.)[10]

Since the 1960s, when family farms began to disappear in the United States, industries that made the components for these high-calorie, processed foods had government subsidies (processed cereal grains, soybeans, livestock, etc.), while fruit and vegetable industries in general have not. Thus fruit and vegetable prices have increased by about 50 percent from 1982 to 2008, with much less marketing of their health benefits to the public. The other food components of the processed food industry that added extra calories and reduced protective micronutrients to our foods have actually had a reduction in real costs. Adjusted for inflation, prices decreased by 10 percent for fats and oils, 15 percent for sugars and sweets, and 34 percent for carbonated soft drinks.[11] Therefore, the public consumes more calories and unhealthy foods because of price, convenience, and lack of knowledge. Do you ever wonder why fast food can be sold for such cheap prices?

The culmination of these five dietary patterns over the last century has led to an unhealthy and devastating food intake pattern in the United States, in which 12 percent of the calorie intake is from plant foods (up to half of which may be processed), 25 percent animal foods (almost all of which is factory farmed, not free-range drug-free animals), and 63 percent processed foods containing added fats, oils, sugars, and refined grains.[12]

U.S. FOOD CONSUMPTION
AS A % OF CALORIES

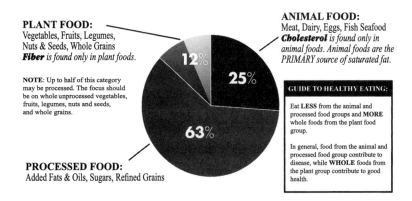

PLANT FOOD:
Vegetables, Fruits, Legumes, Nuts & Seeds, Whole Grains
Fiber is found only in plant foods.

NOTE: Up to half of this category may be processed. The focus should be on whole unprocessed vegetables, fruits, legumes, nuts and seeds, and whole grains.

ANIMAL FOOD:
Meat, Dairy, Eggs, Fish Seafood
Cholesterol is found only in animal foods. Animal foods are the PRIMARY source of saturated fat.

GUIDE TO HEALTHY EATING:

Eat **LESS** from the animal and processed food groups and **MORE** whole foods from the plant food group.

In general, food from the animal and processed food group contribute to disease, while **WHOLE** foods from the plant group contribute to good health.

PROCESSED FOOD:
Added Fats & Oils, Sugars, Refined Grains

Special thanks to Joel Fuhrman, MD, and Amie Hamlin, Executive Director of The New York Coalition for Healthy School Food for permission to reproduce and modify this illustration. Original concept by Joel Fuhrman, MD, in *Eat to Live* (Drfuhrman.com). Graphic design by Michelle Bando (Michellebando.com) as seen at Healthyschoolfood.org/nutrition101.htm, copyright 2009.

Worldwide per capita calorie availability has increased in developing countries since the 1970s, occurring concurrently with increased consumption of meats and animals foods; increased added fats and oils; increased added calorie sweeteners; a mild increase in grain consumption with a decrease in the overall share of grain consumed compared to other foodstuffs; and, a reduction in physical activity. Consequently, chronic diseases are occurring in developing countries at alarming rates as their traditional diets change to more urbanized or "Westernized" diets and daily physical activity is reduced, similar to developed countries.[13]

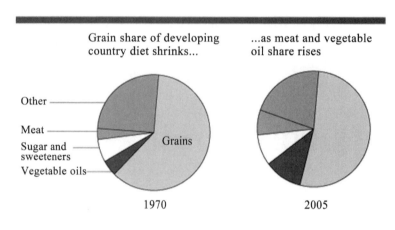

Grain share of developing country diet shrinks... ...as meat and vegetable oil share rises

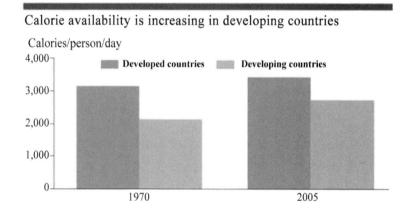

Calorie availability is increasing in developing countries

Source: Food and Agriculture Organization of the United Nations.

Obesity and overweight conditions, derived from modern-day excess calorie consumption and lack of physical activity, lead to many of these chronic conditions. A reduction in excess calorie consumption with an increase in nutrient-dense foods would lead to weight normalization and significantly reduce the incidence of many chronic diseases. This would dramatically reduce healthcare costs and human suffering, while increasing work productivity. Nutrient-dense foods have many health promoting compounds (antioxidants, vitamins, minerals, phytochemicals, fiber, etc.) that are protective against chronic disease progression and can help reverse some of these conditions.

The Simple Solution: The TRIAD Wellness Program

The solution to the modern urbanized lifestyle and ensuing chronic disease is the same for developed and developing countries: practicing simple diet and lifestyle principles, which successful aging populations from around the world have practiced for hundreds of years as part of their normal way of living. While the culture and location of these aging populations is different, the essence of their basic lifestyles is very similar and is generally included in the *9 Simple Steps to Optimal Health* using the **TRIAD Wellness Program**.

For Who and When

The **TRIAD Wellness Program** can be practically applied to the individual, the family, your community, your country, and the world.

Now is the time for this approach because:

- Healthcare in the United States and around the world needs **real reform** from the current disease-care models to prevention-oriented models.

- The current science supports the *Staying Healthy in the Fast Lane* concepts.

- Examples of healthy aging cultures support this approach to healthful living and aging.
- Individuals have used this approach in very busy lifestyles and have maintained a high level of wellness and function.
- The world is busy, aging, and urbanizing rapidly, so it is imperative to implement simple principles and practices that everyone can employ to reduce ever-escalating healthcare costs, loss of work productivity and function, and human suffering that occur from chronic diseases. If we can prevent and reverse chronic disease as individuals and a world community, then we can focus on the pressing and complex world problems that need our attention now.

Changing Food Consumption Patterns in the United States Over the Last Century

Calorie Availability and Consumption Patterns Over The Last 100 Years

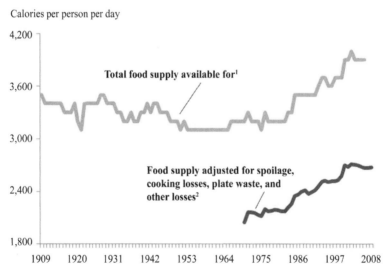

[1]Source: USDA, Centers for Nutrition Policy and Promotion, Nutrient Content of the Food Supply Data based on USDA, Economic Research Service's Food Availability Data. Rounded to the nearest hundred.
[2]Source: USDA, Economic Research Service, Loss-Adjusted Food Availability Data.

Meat Consumption Patterns In The United States Over The Last 100 Years

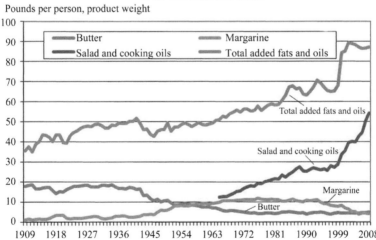

Boneless, trimmed (edible) weight equivalent.
Source: USDA, Economic Research Service, Food Availability Data.

Fats and Oil Consumption Patterns in the United States Over The Last 100 Years

Note: In 2000, the number of firms reporting vegetable oil production increased.
Source: USDA/Economic Research Service estimate using data from Census Bureau.

Calorie Sweetener Consumption Patterns in the United States Over The Last 100 Years

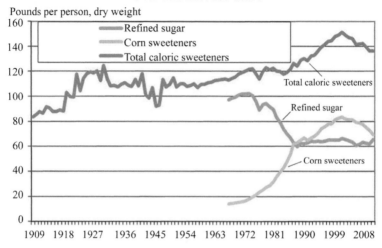

Total caloric sweeteners include refined sugar, corn sweeteners, honey, and other edible syrups.
Source: USDA, Economic Research Service, Food Availability Data.

Cheese Consumption Patterns in the United States Over The Last 100 Years

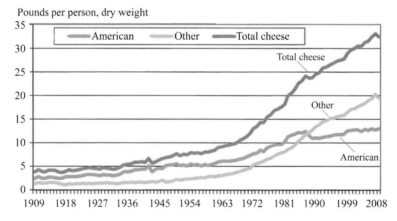

Source: USDA, Economic Research Service, Food Availability Data.

Flour and Cereal Product Consumption Patterns in the United States Over The Last 100 Years

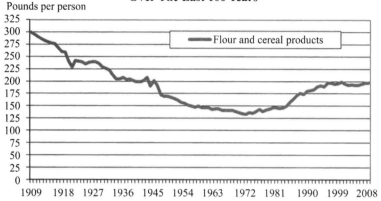

Source: USDA, Economic Research Service, Food Availability Data.
The six above U.S. dietary pattern illustrations were created with the assistance from: Hodan Farah Wells, PhD, economist, Economic Research Service, USDA, hfarah@ers.usda. gov; and Jean Buzby, PhD, agricultural economist with the Economic Research Service, USDA, jbuzby@ers.usda.gov. Source: USDA, Economic Research Service, Food Availability Data.

How Americans Consume Their Grains

Americans eat their whole grains as:

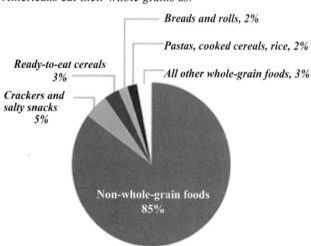

Source: ERS analysis of 1999-2000 National Health and Nutrition Examination Survey (NHANES) data.

U.S. FOOD CONSUMPTION
AS A % OF CALORIES

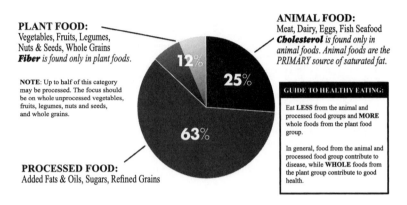

PLANT FOOD:
Vegetables, Fruits, Legumes,
Nuts & Seeds, Whole Grains
Fiber *is found only in plant foods.*

NOTE: Up to half of this category
may be processed. The focus should
be on whole unprocessed vegetables,
fruits, legumes, nuts and seeds,
and whole grains.

ANIMAL FOOD:
Meat, Dairy, Eggs, Fish Seafood
Cholesterol *is found only in
animal foods. Animal foods are the
PRIMARY source of saturated fat.*

GUIDE TO HEALTHY EATING:

Eat **LESS** from the animal and
processed food groups and **MORE**
whole foods from the plant food
group.

In general, food from the animal and
processed food group contribute to
disease, while **WHOLE** foods from
the plant group contribute to good
health.

PROCESSED FOOD:
Added Fats & Oils, Sugars, Refined Grains

12%
25%
63%

Special thanks to Joel Fuhrman, MD, and Amie Hamlin, Executive Director of The New York Coalition for Healthy School Food for permission to reproduce and modify this illustration. Original concept by Joel Fuhrman, MD, in *Eat to Live* (Drfuhrman.com). Graphic design by Michelle Bando (Michellebando.com) as seen at Healthyschoolfood.org/nutrition101.htm, copyright 2009.

Chapter 2

THE AMERICAN LIFESTYLE

Every day my patients tell me that their health and well-being are out of synch with the pace of modern life. Chances are that you, too, share some of their complaints. Think of the last time you told yourself or someone else:

- "I don't have time to exercise."
- "It's too expensive and takes too long to prepare healthy foods."
- "I am too tired to cook; we have to eat out!"
- "There is no time left to take care of me after my family."
- "If I had known getting old was like this, I would have taken better care of myself."
- "These golden years aren't so golden."

It's true that our fast-paced existence has a strong and often negative impact on our health and that we would all feel much better if we could somehow just slow down. It's also true that healthcare costs are skyrocketing and that families and communities across the nation are suffering under a financial burden that will only get worse as the baby boomers move into old age. The *Age Wave*, as visionary psychologist and gerontologist Dr. Ken Dychtwald so aptly calls it, is reaching tsunami proportions and will change the face of healthcare and our economy as the boomers demand more services for the epidemic of chronic diseases with which they will have to live.[1]

The fact is that society isn't likely to change any time soon. If we want to beat the exhaustion-chronic disease cycle, then we as individuals need to find a way to take charge and stay healthy in this rapidly paced modern world. If we want to avoid the crippling costs of twenty-first-century medical care, then we must be willing to honestly assess the choices we are making in our everyday lives and start taking our health into our own hands today. If we do this, we will achieve real and lasting healthcare reform.

Sobering Facts

In John Robbins' must-read book *Healthy at 100* (2007), a few sentences put our present societal health predicament into focus:

> "*A century ago, the average adult in Western nations spent only 1 percent of his or her life in a morbid or ill state, but today's average modern adult spends more than 10 percent of his or her life sick...Throughout the industrialized world, people are living longer but they are getting sick sooner, so the number of years they spend chronically ill is actually increasing in both directions.*"[2]

This next excerpt from *Healthy at 100* made me do a double take since my siblings and I had recently taken care of our mother with chronic, life-ending pulmonary fibrosis. "*...the average twenty-first-century American will likely spend more years caring for parents than for children.*"[3] My siblings and I had more than adequate resources and a great family unit to take care of my mother and keep her at home, but it was hard and time consuming. I can't imagine other families with fewer resources, or individuals with no family at all, and what kind of care they might receive.

These facts, and my experience with my mother and seeing patients and families over the years, drive me to stay as healthy as I can so I can remain independent as I age and not be a burden to my daughter and society.

The Big Problem: Chronic Diseases

As mentioned in Chapter 1, chronic diseases such as heart disease, cancer, high blood pressure, stroke, diabetes, chronic lung, kidney and liver diseases, Parkinson's and Alzheimer's diseases, and diabetes account for 70 percent of all deaths in the United States.[4] These diseases are predominantly caused—and can be prevented—by diet and lifestyle choices. So how have we come to the extreme state of widespread ill health that we are experiencing today?

In 1970, the average adult consumed five hundred fewer calories per day and weighed 19.8 pounds less than in 2000. Similarly, a child in 1970 consumed 350 calories less per day and weighed 8.8 pounds less than in 2000. The numbers don't lie. They perfectly predict our obesity epidemic.[5]

Being Overweight: The Proverbial Elephant in the Room

It is very easy to see when one looks back over the last century in the United States why being overweight, obesity, and inflammatory diseases are becoming more prevalent. The answers are simple: As modern society urbanizes and people's lives center around cities, people become busier; more processed, high-calorie, and prepared foods are made available; and people eat out more frequently.

American households spend more than 40 percent of their total food budget on foods prepared outside of the home, up from 25 percent in 1970.[6] This is problematic because, when we eat at restaurants and fast-food restaurants, we not only consume more food, but we also eat foods with higher caloric density (i.e., added fats and oils, calorie sweeteners, cheeses, meats, refined grains). Furthermore, even the foods we eat at home now tend to be more calorie dense and less nutritionally dense than they were even a few decades ago. For the average person, eating one meal away from home each week equals approximately a two-pound weight gain each year.[7]

These trends, along with a marked decrease in physical activity, can lead to only one thing: increased weight—and lots of it. The good news is that after a quarter-century of increases, obesity prevalence has not measurably increased in the past few years. The bad news is that obesity levels are still high: 34 percent of U.S. adults aged twenty and over. There is a greater percentage of Americans overweight than obese (34.2 percent vs. 33.8 percent). In addition, we now have a new weight category—the extremely obese (> 40 BMI) at 5.7 percent of the population (overweight > 25 BMI; obese >30 BMI).[8] If you add these totals up, over 70 percent of the U.S. population has an excess weight problem!

Trends in Overweight, Obesity, and Extreme Obesity Among Adults Aged 20-74 Years: United States, 1960-2008

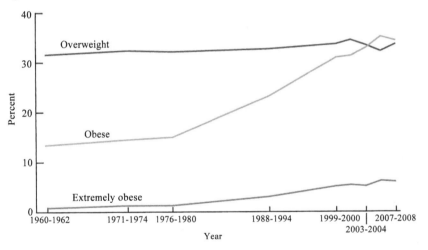

NOTE: Age-adjusted by the direct method to the year 2000 U.S. Census Bureau estimates, using the age groups 20-39, 40-59, and 60-74 years. Pregnant females were excluded. Overweight is defined as a body mass index (BMI) of 25 or greater but less than 30; obesity is a BMI greater than or equal to 30; extreme obesity is a BMI greater than or equal to 40.
SOURCE: CDC/NCHS, National Health Examination Survey cycle I (1960-1962); National Health and Nurition Examination Survey I (1971-1974), II (1976-1980), and III (1988-1994), 1999-2000, 2001-2002, 2003-2004, 2005-2006, and 2007-2008.
Cynthia Ogden and Margaret Carroll, *Prevalence of Overweight, Obesity, and Extreme Obesity Among Adults: United States, Trends 1976–1980 Through 2007–2008*. Division of Health and Nutrition Examination Surveys, National Center for Health Statistics, Centers for Disease Control and Prevention.

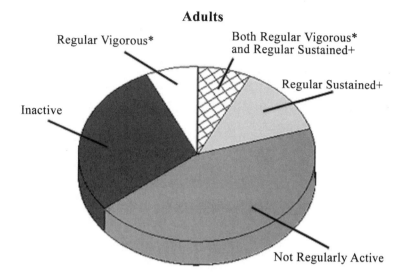

Adults

*Regular Vigourous - 20 minutes 3 times per week of vigorous intensity
+Regular Sustained - 30 minutes 5 times per week of any intensity
SOURCE: CDC 1992 Behavioral Risk Factor Survey.
Physical Activity and Health: A Report From the Surgeon General. Adults. Facts. Centers for Disease Control and Prevention, National Center for Chronic Disease Prevention and Health Promotion.

Being overweight and obesity increase the risks for the following diseases in adults:[9]

- Hypertension (high blood pressure)
- Dyslipidemia (for example, high total cholesterol or high levels of triglycerides)
- Type 2 diabetes
- Coronary heart disease
- Stroke
- Liver and gallbladder disease
- Osteoarthritis (a degeneration of cartilage and its underlying bone within a joint)
- Sleep apnea and respiratory problems
- Some cancers (endometrial, breast, and colon)
- Gynecological problems (abnormal menses, infertility)

The Threat to our Children

Our youth are also experiencing an epidemic of obesity and overweight issues. In total, there has been a tripling of the obesity rate in children since the 1970s. In the age groups of six- to eleven- and twelve- to nineteen-year-olds there has been almost a quadrupling of the obesity rates since the mid-1960s.[10]

These startling obesity and overweight rates, in conjunction with reduced physical activity, explain the even more alarming trends we are starting to recognize, such as an increasing prevalence of type 2 diabetes—a disease of adults—in our youth. And that's just diabetes. The big picture is that the overweight epidemic is putting our youth in the position to develop the same chronic diseases that plague our adult population. The only difference is that they will be getting these diseases at an earlier age than we have ever seen and with more severe consequences. That means living with these diseases longer and costing us a lot more in time, money, and reduced function and productivity.[11] This is the first time ever in American history that children may have a shorter life expectancy than their parents.[12]

Why Have Overweight Issues Dramatically Risen in our Young Children and Teens?

The reasons are pretty much common sense. For one thing, children eat like their parents, who are getting fatter, not thinner. Also, parents are busier, which means less oversight, less patience, less energy, and more dietary shortcuts and junk foods eaten in or out of the house. The calorie-dense processed foods that are available to adults are also available to kids. In addition to the excess calorie exposure that occurs with their parents, kids today are not getting enough physical activity. They spend more time engaging in sedentary technology-based entertainment. Children today are more stressed out than ever before (just like their parents).

Trends in Obesity Among Children and Adolescents: United States, 1963-2008

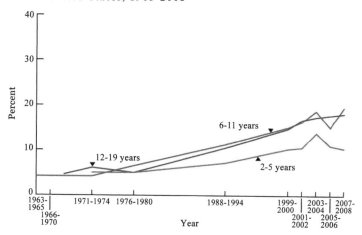

NOTE: Obesity is defined as body mass index (BMI) greater than or equal to sex- and age-specific 95th percentile from the 2000 CDC Growth Charts.
SOURCES: CDC/NCHS, National Examination Surveys II (ages 6-11), III (ages 12-17), and National Health and Nutrition Examination Survey (NHANES) I-III, and NHANES 1999-2000, 2001-2002, 2003-2004, 2005-2006, and 2007-2008.
Cynthia Ogden and Margaret Carroll, *Prevalence of Obesity Among Children and Adolescents: United States, Trends 1963–1965 Through 2007–2008*. Division of Health and Nutrition Examination Surveys, National Center for Health Statistics, Centers for Disease Control and Prevention.

Physical Activity Levels of Adolescents and Young Adults, by Age and Sex

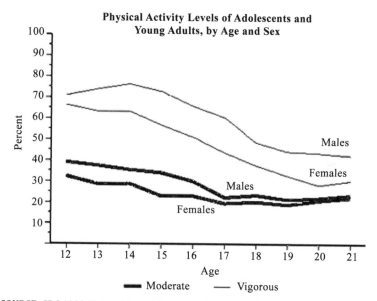

SOURCE: CDC 1992 National Health Interview Survey Youth Risk Behavior Survey
Physical Activity Levels of Adolescents and Young Adults, by Age and Sex. Physical Activity and Health: A Report From The Surgeon General. Centers for Disease Control and Prevention, National Center for Chronic Disease Prevention and Health Promotion.

Our Diet and Lifestyle Cause Inflammation

We are not only consuming excess calories but also a diet that promotes inflammation and leads to all chronic *inflammatory* diseases. This means that the foods we eat—and the portions and combinations in which we eat them—are causing our bodies to exist in a constant state of inflammation that leads to the symptoms and diseases from which we suffer needlessly. The changes that negatively impact our health and well-being are not random or mysterious. They can be traced directly to changes in lifestyles—specifically diet and physical activity choices we have adopted over the course of the last fifty to one hundred years.

These critical U.S. lifestyle changes over the *last century* mentioned in Chapter 1 are worth repeating. They include:

- An increase in total meat consumption[13]
- A dramatic increase in added fats and oils[14]
- Increases in calorie sweeteners (sugar from beet or cane and high fructose corn sweeteners)[15]
- A dramatic increase in cheese consumption[16]
- A decrease in total cereal grains and increase in refined grains[17]
- Reduced physical activity[18]

We simply reverse these diet and lifestyle patterns and we dramatically improve America's health (and prosperity!). At the same time we make these changes, we will create real healthcare reform and this current political debate regarding healthcare becomes non-existent.

Does an Anti-inflammatory Diet and Lifestyle Exist?

We have a problem with chronic diseases that are caused by inflammation. Inflammation is a natural response to stress, infection, injury, and trauma and is a needed response. If inflammation is chronically activated, it leads to a continued release of chemical compounds by the body originally meant to be of short duration that can cause chronic tissue damage and the aforementioned diseases.[19] Excess calories, chronically high blood sugars, low nutrient-dense diets, overweight conditions, and sedentary lifestyles all increase inflammation. We need to reverse these conditions on a daily basis to reverse or slow chronic disease problems. We need to create an anti-inflammatory lifestyle.[20]

Key components of an anti-inflammatory lifestyle, which we will discuss in detail in the "How To" of the **TRIAD Wellness Program,** are:

- Eating *whole unprocessed* foods, especially plant foods, with or without small amounts of foods from animal origin
- Eating lots of *nutrient-dense* unprocessed plant foods
- Avoiding foods to which we are sensitive
- Controlling blood sugar (and insulin)—eating *low glycemic* foods
- Staying *lean*
- Getting daily *physical activity*
- Reducing and/or blending with chronic *stress*

The Bottom Line

Chronic inflammatory diseases plague Western industrialized societies and are now becoming prevalent in developing countries, straining economies and workforces and taxing the healthcare budgets of the world community.[21] Food is the major cause of inflammation. Chronic inflammation causes chronic diseases. Change the types of foods you eat and you can reverse inflammation and chronic diseases individually, locally, nationally, and worldwide. When I collectively look at medical studies, successfully aging cultures, and years of experiencing diseases improved by diet change, it is easy for me to say that *"food is the most powerful medicine there is!"* Two other important causes of inflammation in the modern lifestyle are lack of physical activity and chronically activated mental stress.

Before we get to the "how" of changing this negative health direction, I think it is important to address this next question: Is it just crazy, stressed-out Americans who are struggling with these health issues of chronic disease, or is the rest of the world struggling with these issues as well?

Chapter 3

GLOBAL HEALTH: WHERE ARE WE GOING?

The more I learned about the state of health and chronic disease in North America and developed countries, the clearer it became that over-consumption and lack of physical activity are no longer confined to the wealthiest countries. Data from the World Health Organization (WHO) clearly shows that chronic disease is an increasingly global problem. In fact, the WHO states that 60 percent of deaths are caused by chronic diseases[1]; the major risk factors for chronic disease are an unhealthy diet, physical inactivity, and tobacco use[2]; and *if the major risk factors for chronic disease were eliminated, at least 80 percent of heart disease, stroke, and type 2 diabetes would be prevented and 40 percent of cancer would be prevented.*[3]

As the world "urbanizes" and economies rapidly grow—such as in India, China, and other parts of Asia and Africa—people in these societies start taking on the Western lifestyle. As these populations move from their agrarian rural lifestyle, which was more physically active and predominantly plant based, with whole foods and small amounts of free-range animal foods, their per capita calorie consumption increases. With this increase in calories and reduction in nutrient dense foods and physical activity, come the overweight issues and subsequent chronic diseases of the industrialized countries.

Just as in the United States, the typical diets of developing nations are now characterized by a significant increase in total calories, animal foods (meats), added fats, oils, caloric sweeteners, and a mild increase in grains (but a *reduction* in the percent of calories from grains compared to other food stuffs), in conjunction with a more sedentary lifestyle. In fact, the similarities between the unhealthy trends in Western and developing societies are startling but make sense.[4]

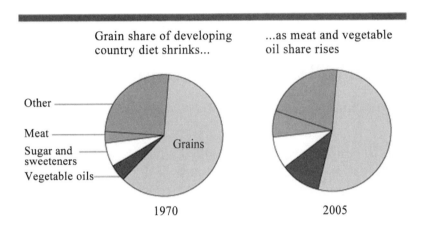

Source: Food and Agriculture Organization of the United Nations.

Why is it important for us to consider the global scope of this problem even before embarking upon our own journey of personal wellness and change? Because everything we do has a ripple effect; every choice we make has ramifications that we may not have ever imagined. If we realize that the patterns of how we, as individuals and societies, live and eat really do affect the rest of the world, then we can make choices that support the production and consumption of healthful food from which people can make a healthy living. At the same time, these healthy choices can preserve the ecological balance of other species on the planet, which eventually effects our survival.

Major Killers Go Global!

As noted by the Economic Research Service of the USDA, "despite the persistence of food insecurity, food consumption has been rising in many developing countries, and with it has come higher rates of being overweight and obesity...."[5]

The WHO projects that by 2015, approximately 2.3 billion adults will be overweight, or about 30 percent of the world's population; and more than 700 million will be obese, or about 10 percent of the world's population. Initially this appeared to be only a problem in high-income countries, but now being overweight and obese are dramatically occurring in low- and middle-income countries, particularly in *urban settings*.[6] Being overweight and obese greatly increases the risk of many of the world's leading disease-related killers. These are listed below.[7]

- Cardiovascular disease, which includes heart disease and stroke, is already the number one killer in the world, killing 17 million people annually.
- Diabetes, which is becoming a global epidemic, will increase by more than 50 percent worldwide in the next ten years.
- Some cancers, including endometrial, breast, and colon.
- Musculoskeletal disorders, especially osteoarthritis.

Furthermore, childhood obesity is associated with a higher chance of premature death and disability in adulthood.[8]

These statistics point to a crisis situation. Many low-income countries are now facing a double burden of risk: They continue to deal with problems of infectious disease and under-nutrition at the same time that they are experiencing a rapid upsurge in chronic diseases related to excess calories from more processed and animal-based foods. It is now common for under-nutrition and obesity to exist side by side within the same country.[9]

Let's look a bit more closely at these leading killers and at the impact they are having around the world in order to gain a better understanding of the true scope of this problem.

Heart Disease

Heart disease, which is still the number one cause of death worldwide (cancer may overtake heart disease this year), is becoming a terrible problem in countries with rapidly developing economies such as India and China, and in Japan, where they continue to develop a more urban lifestyle similar to that of the United States.

The Asia Pacific Cohort Studies Collaboration analyzed data from six hundred thousand people involved in forty-three studies in nine places: China, Hong Kong, Thailand, Singapore, Australia, Japan, South Korea, Taiwan, and New Zealand. Findings from this exhaustive body of research show conclusively that "Asia is facing a cardiovascular disease epidemic as a result of increases in obesity, high blood pressure, and smoking."[10]

India, too, is being overwhelmed by heart disease. In fact, India now carries 60 percent of the world's heart disease burden, with the same risk factors as elsewhere.[11]

Cancer

Cancer alone accounted for approximately 13 percent of worldwide deaths in 2007, or 7.9 million people. Nearly 72 percent of these cancer deaths occurred in low- and middle-income countries, where leading risk factors include low fruit and vegetable intake in addition to tobacco and alcohol use and infections from hepatitis B and C and the human papilloma virus. In high-income countries, where infectious disease is rarer, being overweight or obese, coupled with tobacco and alcohol use, are the primary causes of cancer.[12]

Diabetes

The WHO estimates that more than 220 million people worldwide have diabetes. This number is likely to exceed 366 million by the year 2030.[13]

In general, diabetes is a chronic disease in which the cells do not absorb sugar efficiently to be used as energy, and subsequently blood sugar and insulin rise. Both can have adverse consequences on health. There are three primary types of diabetes: type 1, type 2, and gestational diabetes. There is also a fourth abnormal blood sugar condition called pre-diabetes.

- Type 1 diabetes results from the body's failure to produce insulin, the hormone that "unlocks" the cells of the body, from the pancreas, allowing glucose to enter and fuel them. It is estimated that 5 to 10 percent of the world's diabetics have type 1 diabetes. This is the type that usually occurs in children. It requires insulin to be administered in conjunction with diet and exercise.[14]

- Type 2 diabetes is the most common form of diabetes in the United States and worldwide, accounting for about 85 to 95 percent of all diabetics. Type 2 diabetes results from insulin resistance (a condition in which the body fails to properly use insulin), combined with relative insulin deficiency. Though there is a genetic component, and there may be environmental pollutants and abnormal microflora that increase the development of type 2 diabetes, this condition is very much associated with excess weight and calories and a sedentary lifestyle. Type 2 diabetes occurs more frequently with aging. This form of diabetes is predominantly a lifestyle disease and can be *prevented* and *reversed* with aggressive lifestyle management.[15]

- Gestational diabetes is the high blood sugar (hyperglycemia) that occurs during pregnancy. It may be caused by hormones released during pregnancy that inhibit insulin's actions.

- These individuals after pregnancy may be more susceptible to type 2 diabetes.[16]
- Pre-diabetes is a condition affecting 57 million Americans, or about 19 percent of the U.S. population. It is a state of chronic blood sugar elevation just under the definition of diabetes (a fasting blood sugar between 100 and 125 mg/dl). The adverse consequences of elevated blood sugar to the blood vessels, nerves, eyes, and other organs are still occurring in this "pre-diabetic" state.[17]

The WHO estimates that without urgent action, diabetic deaths will increase globally by more than 50 percent in the next ten years and over 80 percent in upper-middle-income countries by 2015.[18]

Cardiovascular Disease

Cardiovascular disease is the number one cause of death globally. By 2030, more than 23 million people will die annually from cardiovascular disease, many from heart disease and stroke. Cardiovascular diseases are still projected to remain the single leading cause of death in 2030.[19]

The causes of cardiovascular disease are well known. They include unhealthy diets and physical inactivity, which can result in high blood pressure, high blood glucose, high blood fats, being overweight, and obese. These are called intermediate risk factors. The major modifiable risk factors are unhealthy diet, physical inactivity, and tobacco use. These risk factors can account for approximately 80 percent of coronary heart disease and cerebrovascular disease.[20]

On paper, all three of these major chronic diseases (cancer, diabetes, and heart disease) are simple to change. There is no magical medical breakthrough needed here, no magical new supplements needed—just those *9 Simple Steps to Optimal Health.*

Economic and Societal Costs of Chronic Disease

Chronic diseases associated with the Westernization of global diet and lifestyle affect many people in middle age. Very often, this creates severe financial hardship for individuals and their families; in turn, lost earnings and out-of-pocket healthcare payments undermine the socioeconomic development of communities and nations.

Consider the fact that by the year 2050, the world's elderly population—people age sixty years and older—will have more than tripled from 600 million (in the year 2000) to 2 billion.[21] Good health is essential so that older people can maintain their independence and participation in family and community life. Good functional health is also important in the elderly to reduce the healthcare costs and resources needed from local and national economies, which will be severely strained by these aging populations.

The Crux of the Dilemma

A difficult concept to grasp is the juxtaposition of overweight issues and excess calories with under-nutrition in impoverished settings. Excess calories can keep people alive—at least for a while. But if they are "empty" calories—not attached to vitamins, minerals, fatty acids, fiber, and protective phytochemicals—then they offer little protection from the chronic diseases that are killing us.

Most Americans think we are the best-nourished people in the world because we are big and strong (and fat). Yes and no. It's true we have more access to foodstuffs and food calories than most people do. But if we spend our time buying quick, highly processed refined foods, we get a whole lot of calories without beneficial nutrients, and we get fat and/or develop chronic diseases. The health problem and solution are the same for all economic strata in urban settings: The "haves" of the world must educate and discipline themselves to eat low-calorie, nutrient-dense foods and exercise. The "haves" need to use modern-day technology to their advantage to enhance their access to whole foods and to places where they can get adequate daily physical activity while living very busy lifestyles. We must also work to help those in lower economic situations to have access to whole foods at a reasonable cost and to change their belief systems. The new, modern-day diet of highly processed, high calorie-dense, and low nutrient-dense foods is not really progress at all or healthful. (Rather, the "old" ways of eating whole, unprocessed foods that are closer to the ground are much better.) Eating less is usually eating more healthfully. Also, physical labor is healthy, and if people aren't getting any, they need to.

Part II:

The Solution

Chapter 4

PREVENTIVE CARE VS. DISEASE CARE: CHANGING THE PARADIGM

Efforts at healthcare reform are doomed to failure unless we switch from a disease care model to a preventive one. The only way healthcare can be sustainable in this country and around the world is for people to live lifestyles that prevent chronic disease—period! No healthcare system can withstand the cost of chronic disease treatment and management that will inevitably continue to grow with a rapidly aging population. We must turn our *disease care model* into a *preventive care model* to be affordable and sustainable.

The problem is that the economic incentives and political forces to do this will be very difficult to change. No matter how well intentioned, I'm not sure any administration or government can change these competing forces, *but I do know that* **you** *can change, making the above political dilemma a moot point.*

It's all on you! You can make yourself healthy by just doing the *9 Simple Steps* daily and consistently. You cannot lose. It's not dependent on the stock market or your boss—just *you.* And truly, there is nothing more straightforward with a one-to-one response of *effort to results* than applying these steps to your health.

Americans could dramatically reduce occurrence of chronic disease, solve the healthcare crisis, and increase national productivity within months with these simple, cost-effective changes in lifestyle. A simple five-food-group diet of vegetables, fruit, beans, nuts and seeds, and whole grains—with minimal or no animal products (plus exercise)—can create this dramatic change.

A recent example of this in your average, hard-working American was the use of a low-fat vegan (animal-free) diet among GEICO employee volunteers who were obese and/or had a previous diagnosis of type 2 diabetes. After a twenty-two-week worksite research study on this diet, there was a reduction in body weight of more than eleven pounds and waist circumference reduction of more than two inches.[1] Another practical example of applying a "plant-strong" dietary approach in the real world has been demonstrated by Rip Esselstyn, triathlete, health advocate, author of *The Engine 2 Diet* (2009), and Texas fireman. Rip has shown how well this diet and lifestyle approach works in reducing weight and cardiovascular risk in a hard-working, all-American fireman in the heart of Texas. If it can be done in this setting, it can be done anywhere. You may say you don't want to make these diet and lifestyle changes. Fine, but don't blame the government or anyone else for spiraling healthcare costs! **It's all on you** once you are educated.

After the country is "lean and fit," if you have to add in some animal foods, then you can do it, though I don't recommend it. Healthy aging cultures do not eat as much animal foods as Americans do, and when they do, they don't eat mass-produced, factory-farm animals. Virtually none of these "Blue Zone" or "Cold Spot" healthy aging societies eat the highly processed, high-fat, high-sugar, and highly refined grain diets that we do as well. ("Blue Zones" refer to places where chronic diseases are low and people live long, functional lives. A "Cold Spot" is an area where a specific chronic disease occurs very infrequently or not at all.)

The bottom line is that it's your choice to live an unhealthy lifestyle once you are educated on the basics of health. After you read this book, you will have that simple, basic knowledge, and you'll have simple daily steps to make this happen in the busy, modern world—quickly! The kind of change I am talking about is not only possible but also simple, affordable, and can even be fun. I've seen others do it; so can you!

There will always be an exception to every rule. A small minority of people might not feel well applying these principles initially. Still, if you follow the guidelines presented in this book and remember nothing else but these *9 Simple Steps to Optimal Health,* the vast majority of you will be more healthy and more in control of your own health.

No society can function efficiently in the long run with any devised healthcare system if it has a predominantly disease care model in which you let disease happen—especially the chronic diseases mentioned here repeatedly—and then try to treat them with pharmaceuticals and surgery as your main medical approaches. Prevention and treatment by diet, exercise, and lifestyle have to be the mainstays of any healthcare delivery system.

The U.S. healthcare model is absolutely backward. Until some real incentive comes for keeping people well—or unless people themselves see the light—things won't change. Healthcare costs will continue to spiral. There will be more drugs prescribed, more disability and suffering, and more loss of national economic productivity.

Let's get on with how to create the best health insurance we can: a self-managed wellness lifestyle that will dramatically reduce these chronic diseases and allow us to control our health destiny if we choose to.

Chapter 5

THE GOOD NEWS: CHRONIC DISEASE IS PREVENTABLE AND REVERSIBLE

According to the WHO, there is ample evidence that we are taking part in...

> "...a global shift in diet toward increased intake of energy-dense foods that are high in fat and sugars, but low in vitamins, minerals, and other micronutrients; and a trend towards decreased physical activity due to increasingly sedentary nature of many forms of work, changing modes of transportation and increasing urbanization."[1]

The state of global health would change immediately for the better if we were to follow the above *reworded "health-positive"* statement:

> *We are choosing* a global shift in diet toward increased intake of *nutrient-dense* foods that are *low* in fat and sugars and *high* in vitamins, minerals, and other micronutrients; and a trend toward *increased* physical activity due to the convenience of many workout facilities in urban environments and work settings, along with employee incentives. *Urbanization provides easier access to a variety of whole, nutrient-dense plant foods, such as vegetables, fruit, beans, nuts, seeds, whole grains, and greater opportunities for exercise.*

Good health is about applying very simple principles on a consistent and daily basis. Fortunately for us, such a transition is not dependent upon new scientific breakthroughs or the creation of brand new social models. All we must do is look to successfully aging cultures, such as the Okinawan centenarians, Nicoyans in Costa Rica, Sardinians in Italy, Seventh Day Adventists in the greater Los Angeles area, and others from around the world—or Blue Zone populations (see *The Blue Zone* by Dan Buettner, 2008). These cultures are examples of the fact that it is possible, practical, and pleasurable to lead healthy and functional lives into advanced age, with reduced chronic disease, if only we would slow down, educate ourselves, and apply some basic principles.

What's a Good Diet?

Top experts in global health agree. In fact, the WHO recommendations on diet are almost exactly the same as the Unified Dietary Guidelines (UDG) outlined by the American Heart Association, American Cancer Society, American Dietetic Association, American Academy of Pediatrics, National Institutes of Health, and American Society of Clinical Nutrition.[2]

WHO Recommendations on Diet
• Achieve energy balance at a healthy weight.
• Limit energy intake from total fats and shift fat consumption away from saturated fat to unsaturated fats and toward the elimination of transfatty acids.
• Increase consumption of fruit and vegetables, legumes, whole grains, and nuts.
• Eliminate the intake of free sugars.
• Limit salt (sodium) consumption from all sources. Use iodized salt.
Global Strategy on Diet, Physical Activity and Health: Diet, World Health Organization. http://www.who.int/dietphysicalactivity/diet/en/index.html (accessed Feb. 26, 2011).

U.S. Unified Dietary Guidelines

- Eat a variety of foods.

- Choose most of what you eat from plant sources.

- Eat five or more servings of fruit and vegetables each day.

- Eat six or more servings of bread, pasta, and cereal grains each day.

- Eat high-fat foods sparingly, especially those from animal sources.

- Keep your intake of simple sugars to a minimum.

Fisher, Edward A., et al., "Summary of a Scientific Conference on Preventive Nutrition: Pediatrics to Geriatrics." *Circulation* 100, (1999):450-456.

"New Unified Dietary Guidelines Offer Nutritional Protection Against Wide Range Of Killer Diseases." *ScienceDaily*. (June 22, 1999). http://www.sciencedaily.com/releases/1999/06/990622061026.htm (accessed June 11, 2011).

Both dietary guidelines recommend eating more fruit and vegetables, more whole grains, and less fat and sugar. Those are big recommendations and would go a long way to safely normalizing weight, which would reduce all chronic diseases. Indirectly, the WHO guidelines encourage fewer animal foods, like the UDG, because animal foods generally have most of the saturated fat and are usually more calorie dense than whole plant foods. In other words, animal foods generally contain more calories per weight or volume than unprocessed plant foods, leading to excess calories, weight gain, and inflammation.

The WHO guidelines are correct in recommending the reduction of trans-fatty acids, which come from confectionary processed foods to extend shelf life, oxidized oils from frying, and margarines. Trans-fatty acids increase cholesterol levels and cardiovascular risk and may alter inflammation and neurologic function by altering cell membrane structure.

Eat Your Fruit and Vegetables

The WHO notes that low fruit and vegetable intake is among the top ten risk factors contributing to death. Up to 2.7 million lives could be saved each year with adequate fruit and vegetable consumption.[3] Americans really have no excuse. Almost all grocery stores have fruit year-round. I know some purists are thinking that we should eat only eat organic fruit and vegetables that are locally grown and in season. I agree—have at it!—but I am thinking of the overall health of my country and the world when I say simply: Eat more fruit and vegetables, whether organic or non-organic, in season or out of season, locally grown or flown in from the Southern Hemisphere, frozen or fresh. Just do it! *Eat at least half of your total food intake as vegetables!*

The WHO Says, "Get Moving!"

According to the WHO, physical inactivity is an independent risk factor for chronic diseases and overall is estimated to cause 1.9 million deaths globally. Physical activity, on the other hand, is fundamental to energy balance and weight control, reduces the risk of coronary heart disease and stroke, reduces the risk of type 2 diabetes, and reduces the risk of some cancers. At least thirty minutes (preferably sixty) of regular, moderately intense physical activity on most days reduces the risk of cardiovascular disease, diabetes, colon cancer, and breast cancer. Muscle strengthening and balance training can reduce falls and increase function in older individuals.[4]

Reducing the Risk of Cancer

Approximately 30 percent of cancers could be prevented by reducing key risk factors, according to an international group of cancer researchers in a 2005 study. Key cancer risk factors are:[5]

- Tobacco use
- Being overweight and/or obese
- Low fruit and vegetable intake
- Physical inactivity
- Alcohol use
- Sexually transmitted infections, such as HIV and HPV
- Urban air pollution
- Indoor smoke from household use of solid fuels
- Sunlight exposure

Generally, the WHO perspectives on health are excellent, but I would exercise caution in recommending the *complete* avoidance of sunlight on a mass scale. Sunlight is a critical nutrient and a health-promoting agent. In fact, it is probably a lifesaver if used properly and could cheaply and effectively improve the world's health the way few, if any, approaches could.

The cancers of the skin that arise from excessive or improper sun exposure (squamous or basal cell cancers) are generally not as lethal, with squamous cell causing more deaths (2,500 deaths per year) than basal cell cancers which causes few deaths but can be very disfiguring.[6] Melanoma, the most life-threatening form of skin cancer, accounts for 75 percent of all deaths from skin cancer while providing less than 5 percent of the skin cancer incidence.[7] Melanoma occurs on non-sun-exposed areas of the body as well as sun-exposed.[8] It occurs more frequently in indoor workers than outdoor workers chronically exposed to sunlight.[9] A tan or dark skin, and the ability to tan provides some protection against melanoma.[10] With the use of sunscreens, which predominantly block UVB light needed for protective tanning and the manufacturing of vitamin D, there has been a linear increase, not decrease, in the incidents of melanoma. This may be due to an increase in damaging UVA light that is not blocked by sunscreens generally, as well as increased sun exposure from ignorance of believed sunscreen protection.[11]

Another risk factor for melanoma may be a thick ozone layer (such as in certain parts of Australia), which blocks UVB light, thereby reducing vitamin D synthesis and the production of melanin to darken (protect) the skin, yet allows excessive damaging UVA exposure to occur.[12] Sunlight as the *main cause* of melanomas just doesn't fit consistently.[13] Likewise just using sunscreen to reduce melanoma incidence hasn't worked either.[14]

Moderate and consistent sun exposure (*not burning*) is probably one of the most important preventive health activities in which we can engage to reduce the worldwide instance of cancer, heart disease, high blood pressure, bone loss, depression, and other disorders related to immune function.[15] You don't see the long-living "Blue Zone" cultures staying indoors and avoiding the sun. They aren't sunbathing either, but they are outside doing physical labor such as gardening, farming, herding, fishing, or other necessary work for daily survival. They also eat unprocessed diets that are rich in protective antioxidants and phytochemicals.[16] It is very difficult to get vitamin D from whole-food sources unless you are eating animal livers or whole fish regularly. Generally you get vitamin D from sunlight exposure (the best way, in my opinion), fortified foods (usually not enough), or supplementation (the average person has to do this).

Dermatologists—actually all doctors—should routinely measure (and correct) vitamin D levels for all their patients several times per year and at the time of diagnosis of their cancers. I predict low levels would be found. Vitamin D levels are easy and cheap to correct with supplementation (and/or judicious sun exposure).

I realize sun exposure and skin cancer is a tremendously controversial topic and getting sunburned is not a good thing, but "throwing the baby out with the bath water" with complete sun avoidance and "chemical" protection doesn't make total sense either.[17]

What does make sense to me is to get ten to twenty minutes of sun exposure daily, preferably while doing physical work or exercise. Wear a hat to protect your head and face if you wish. If you can tan get a light tan; DON'T sunburn (especially children);[18] and eat an antioxidant and phytochemical-rich, unrefined, *colorful* plant-based diet that has an array of natural cancer fighting compounds in their natural combinations. Take *at least* 2,000 IU of vitamin D daily and see your dermatologist or skilled primary care physician for a skin exam yearly or biannually. Again, look at the "Blue Zone" cultures that live a long time and don't get cancers in general. They are not housebound and sun avoiders (nor sunbathers) lathering on sunblock. They also don't eat highly processed foods but rather nutrient-dense and antioxidant-rich foods that can protect their skin from sun damage and cancer in general.

Reducing the Diabetic Epidemic

Without urgent action, diabetes-related deaths worldwide will increase by more than 50 percent in the next ten years.[19] To help prevent type 2 diabetes and its complications, people should:[20]

- achieve and maintain a healthy body weight.
- be physically active (at least thirty minutes of regular, moderately intense activity on most days). More physical activity is required for weight control.

The recommendations by the WHO for diabetes reduction are very simple and familiar: normalize weight and get exercise. Ninety to ninety-five percent of diabetes in the United States is type 2 diabetes (five to ten percent type 1).[21] Even though there is a genetic predisposition to type 2 diabetes[22] and there is data relating persistent organic pollutants (POPs)[23] and abnormal gut bacteria to the incidents of diabetes,[24] type 2 diabetes is very much a lifestyle disease that is preventable and treatable, almost always with weight normalization and physical activity. In fact, type 2 diabetes is *reversible* most of the time, and this epidemic need not exist. We should not be using the mindset of "controlling" type 2 diabetes with a little lifestyle change, a lot of medicine, and more research. We should expect the *eradication* of type 2 diabetes by getting lean, physically active, and consuming an unprocessed, whole-food diet that is high in fiber, *low in fat*, and rich in complex carbohydrates from beans, fruit, vegetables, whole grains, small amounts of nuts and seeds, and small amounts of free-ranged animal foods if you think you must eat animal foods (optional, though not recommended). This approach has been proven to normalize weight and lower blood sugar and insulin levels. This unrefined, unprocessed plant-based diet rich in vegetables, beans, fruit, nuts, and seeds, and whole grains (unprocessed carbohydrates) that is very low in fat, is the simplest way to reverse the diabetes epidemic. Therefore, it is the diet of choice for type 2 diabetes.[25]

Eradicating Type 2 Diabetes: The Model for Chronic Disease Reversal?

Diabetes is the epitome of a Western lifestyle disease. It is rapidly treatable with focused diet and lifestyle choices. Type 2 diabetes doesn't need to exist. In fact, type 2 diabetes is rare in cultures in which people eat their traditional, more agrarian, and/or indigenous diets of simple, fresh, local whole foods that have low glycemic indexes and are physically active as a result of manual labor (and they are lean).

Diabetes (Type 2) Reversal Is Possible

Over the last several years, I have had the great privilege of interviewing five of the world's experts on using diet to prevent, slow, and many times reverse diabetes:

- Dr. James W. Anderson, Professor Emeritus, University of Kentucky, founder of the HCF (high carbohydrate, high fiber) diet for diabetes, who has been controlling, preventing, and reversing diabetes for more than thirty years and has published extensively.[26]
- Dr. David Jenkins, MD, PhD, DSc, founder of the famous Glycemic Index and Dietary Portfolio for dramatically lowering cholesterol and improving diabetes.[27]
- Neal Barnard, MD, author of *Dr. Neal Barnard's Program for Reversing Diabetes* (2007) and leading investigator in a National Institute of Health study showing a low-fat, four-food

group, vegan diet has greater benefit in treating diabetes than the conventional ADA diet.[28]

- Dr. Joel Fuhrman, family physician and best-selling author and speaker (*Eat To Live,* 2011, *Eat For Health,* 2008) famous for his concept of consuming the most nutrient-dense foods per calorie for weight control, chronic disease reversal (including diabetes), and optimal health.[29]

- Internist John McDougall, MD, best-selling author and speaker who has been reversing chronic diseases, including diabetes, with low-fat, starch-based diets for more than thirty years. Dr. McDougall is the medical director and founder of the renowned Dr. McDougall's Health and Medical Center and the McDougall Program, a ten-day residential program in Santa Rosa, California.[30]

After spending hours interviewing these five experts and looking at the scientific data, as well as my own patient care experience, I can say unequivocally that most type 2 diabetics could reverse their condition or improve it dramatically if they normalized their weight, became physically active, and ate a predominantly *whole-food, unrefined, low-fat, micronutrient-rich, plant-based* diet with no or minimal animal foods.

If we just took this one chronic disease and followed these physicians' collective advice, which is very similar, we would wipe out this needless diabetes epidemic. With it would go the world's number one killer (heart disease), as well as obesity, and there would also be a significant reduction in cancer with these same lifestyle changes.

This would be real and lasting healthcare reform. No government and corporate "smoke and mirrors" is needed to accomplish this goal. Just an educated and committed you and me. Yes, it is that simple!

The goal of worldwide diabetes (type 2) eradication is a great place to start really changing the world's health. It can be done. First, we have to believe it and envision it; the science and know-how are there. Now we just have to do it.

What about Type 1 Diabetes?

Please don't misinterpret my focus on type 2 diabetes by thinking that I am not concerned about the tragedy of type 1 diabetes, which is more prevalent in children, because it deeply saddens me. Type 1 diabetes is less prevalent than type 2 diabetes, and once it occurs it is not reversible. It accounts for 5 to 15 percent of the total diabetics, depending on what population you study.[31]

The plant-strong diet approach I have been recommending will not cure type 1 diabetes, but it can help control it, many times reducing the level of insulin requirements. Most importantly, the plant-based approach mentioned previously that can dramatically prevent and even reverse type 2 diabetes, helps protect against the consequences of lifelong high blood sugar and insulin levels, such as eye, kidney, nerve, and cardiovascular damage.

While researching new ways to create insulin in the body are important, studying why type 1 diabetes occurs in the first place is equally if not more important. Three areas that I would like to see studied urgently are as follows:

- The role of vitamin D deficiency during pregnancy, lactation, and early childhood, setting the stage for an autoimmune or infectious insult that might damage the pancreas in the first place, leading to lack of insulin production.[32]

- The role of *early* cow's milk and wheat (gluten) introduction in children, triggering an autoimmune reaction resulting in damage to the same insulin-producing cells in the pancreas.[33]

- The role of altered microflora and intestinal immune dysfunction in setting the stage for antigen uptake that results in autoimmune destruction of the insulin-producing cells in the pancreas.[34]

The bottom line is that these three potential causes of type 1 diabetes are so easy to correct if implicated. They can do no harm and may result in lifelong benefit. Take vitamin D during pregnancy and start it immediately after birth in the child; avoid cow's milk products in childhood; and possibly supplement with probiotics during pregnancy, lactation, and throughout childhood. Finding out how to prevent type 1 diabetes by modulation of environmental and dietary factors is critically important and should be a major research focus in diabetic industries and by public health institutions.

Reducing the Burden of Cardiovascular Disease

According to the WHO, at least 80 percent of premature deaths from cardiovascular disease and stroke could be avoided through healthy diet, regular physical activity, and cessation of tobacco use. That means that we can easily and effectively reduce our risk of cardiovascular disease by:[35]

- engaging in regular physical activity,[36]
- avoiding tobacco use and secondhand smoke,[37]
- choosing a diet rich in fruit and vegetables, and avoiding foods that are high in fat, sugar, refined carbohydrates, and salt, and[38]
- maintaining an ideal body weight.[39]

Yet while the WHO recommendations include most of the components of a heart-protective lifestyle, I think they don't go far enough to really reverse heart disease. To profoundly reduce the risk of heart disease, I believe we have to emphasize a dramatic reduction (preferably elimination) in animal-based foods, which includes total meats and dairy products, and encourage the consumption of *only* whole-grain products when grains are consumed. We also need to eliminate added fats, oils, and sugars by eating whole foods only. And of course, eat lots more vegetables, fruit and beans, and small amounts of raw nuts or seeds. The newer version of the American Heart Association's Step I and Step II diet, the Therapeutic Lifestyle Changes (TLC) diet, is better, but probably still not drastic enough to reverse heart disease.[40]

Is Heart Disease Reversible? Yes!

Heart disease reversal by aggressive diet and lifestyle change was shown over thirty years ago by the late Nathan Pritikin and fifty years ago by California cardiologist Dr. Lester Morrison.[41] Within the last twenty years, the excellent work of Dean Ornish, MD, in his landmark 1990 paper in the *Lancet* [42] and in his excellent 1991 book, *Dr. Dean Ornish's Program For Reversing Heart Disease,*[43] has also shown that a very low-fat, unrefined, mainly plant-based diet, with exercise and stress management, can reverse heart disease. Dr. Ornish's work really put the whole concept of a diet and lifestyle approach to reversing heart disease on the road to legitimacy with his published work in the *Lancet.*

In recent years, popular books such as *Stop Inflammation Now* by cardiologist Richard Fleming, MD[44] and *Prevent and Reverse Heart Disease*[45] by internationally recognized surgeon Caldwell B. Esselstyn Jr., MD, (and his son, Rip Esselstyn's, new book, *The Engine 2 Diet*),[46] continue sharing meticulously documented cases of heart disease reversal by very aggressive diet and lifestyle programs with a common modality of whole-food, unrefined, low-fat, plant-based diets that virtually eliminate all animal foods, especially in the early "reversal" phase.

The China Project, one of the most comprehensive databases on the multiple causes of disease ever compiled, was initiated in 1983, and the book *The China Study* (2006), with key investigator and co-author T. Colin Campbell, PhD from Cornell University, showed virtually no heart disease in parts of rural China where cholesterol levels ranged from 90 to 170 mg/dl (average 125 to 130), and the diets of these individuals were predominantly plant-based.[47]

William Castelli, MD, former director of the famed Framingham Heart Study in a recent interview I had with him stated the number of people who have had heart attacks with a cholesterol level below 150 since Framingham's beginning in 1948 was about a half a dozen people. Dr. Castelli said the following when asked if he couldn't use drugs, but he could get the average American to go on the diet of his choice to reverse heart disease, "I would do it (diet) and it would work better than the drugs." He continues,

"Well you'd have them on a pure vegetarian diet and not getting fat on the vegetarian diet." Dr. Castelli commented on two past diet trials that showed reversal of heart disease, the St. Thomas Hospital Study in London and the Dean Ornish Study. "In any event, what we've learned is that in these reversibility trials, that the two diet trials, for the same fall in cholesterol if you get there with diet you did get twice the shrinkage of the deposits than trying to do it with drugs alone." He further comments on the effectiveness of diet therapy for atherosclerosis, "...it's much better if you can get people to go on a diet. Now if I would have put everyone on a vegetarian diet and drive their numbers down by diet, we would get rid of all the atherosclerosis in America." [48]

Dr. Castelli feels to prevent or reverse heart disease from all his years of experience a low fat, unrefined vegetarian diet is best and special attention should be given to keeping one's triglycerides below 60 by reducing all refined carbohydrates, and keeping the total cholesterol:HDL ratio below 3.5. He feels these are the two strongest lipid markers of cardio-protection and have been somewhat over-looked with all the attention given to lowering LDL cholesterol. [49]

The highly honored Cleveland Clinic breast cancer and thyroid/parathyroid surgeon turned heart disease reversal advocate Dr. Caldwell B. Esselstyn Jr. sums up for me the certainty that an aggressive plant-based diet can prevent and reverse heart disease in a recent interview I had with him:

> "...I therefore decided it would be more appropriate to look at the leading killer of women and men in Western civilization, which is cardiovascular disease and heart attacks because in this global research it was very apparent that there were many cultures where heart disease and heart attacks were virtually non-existent. I mean, even today if you're a cardiac surgeon and you go to rural China or the Papua Highlands in New Guinea, or if you go to central Africa or the Tarahumara Indians in northern Mexico, forget it. You'd better plan on selling pencils because you're not going to find cardiovascular disease there, and it's largely because of that plant-based nutrition, and that's what made me feel

that if we could get people to eat to save their hearts they would actually then be saving themselves from cancer as well, and I still think that's true."[50]

The diet and lifestyle principles in any one of the four books mentioned (by Drs. Esselstyn, Ornish, Fleming, and Rip Esselstyn), if applied with diligence, will stop the progression of and reverse heart disease in many people. Heart disease, the world's number one killer, can be relegated to a "toothless paper tiger," as Dr. Esselstyn also stated in his interview with me.[51]

Coincidently, former President Bill Clinton recently switched to an unprocessed plant-based diet before his daughter Chelsea's wedding. This resulted in a dramatic 24 pound weight loss. He did this because he had already had bypass surgery for his heart, his stent had clogged up, and he was influenced by the researchers I have just spoken about (Caldwell Esselstyn, MD; Dean Ornish, MD; and Dr. T. Colin Campbell and son Thomas M. Campbell) and their work on plant-based nutrition reversing heart disease. He shares his reasons and experience with this diet change in a CNN interview with Wolf Blitzer.[52]

While there are a good number of credible health professionals who debate the role of fat and cholesterol reduction in heart disease management—such as cardiologist Stephen Sinatra, MD, who recommends a PAM diet (Pan-Asian Mediterranean diet) of approximately 80 percent plant foods and 20 percent animal foods[53]—the common points in most cardio-protective diets are: eating only unprocessed foods, large portions of plant foods rich in phytochemicals, and a low glycemic diet, which controls blood sugar and insulin and therefore reduces inflammation, the real cause of hardening of the arteries.

You might be wondering why I am taking so much time on type 2 diabetes and heart disease treatment by diet and lifestyle and using the word "reversible." First, I am tired of hearing the words, "Take your medication, eat right, get some exercise, and donate to our society, and we will find a cure in the *near future*." The cure is already here! No more donations and *controlling* diabetes and heart disease. *It is time to get rid of them*. The same diet will greatly reduce the incidence of both. Right now! The "Number One" killer can be eradicated and the epidemic of diabetes stopped. With this will come the dramatic reduction of all chronic diseases and a new, sustainable era in healthcare where low-cost lifestyle changes are the most powerful medicines, and we are free of the self-inflicted shackles of healthcare reform, insurance companies, and pharmaceutical and hospital expenses. It's right there for the taking for every one of us. Read the books and listen to the interviews and references I share if you don't believe me. If you don't want to educate yourself, just do the *9 Simple Steps to Optimal Health* strictly for three to six months and see what happens!

Chronic Disease Prevention and our Children

In order to adequately address the systemic health risks that threaten our children, parents must make a commitment to live and eat differently. Parents must create a lifestyle for the whole family that is centered predominantly on unrefined, nutrient-rich, and less calorie-dense whole plant foods and minimal amounts of processed and animal foods.

Furthermore, we need to become engaged with our schools in order to ensure that they are providing healthy, whole foods (vegetables, fruit, whole grains, beans, nuts, seeds), especially whole-grain products, on their premises. There should also be vegetarian alternatives such as veggie burgers and chili, marinara sauces, and the like. When I say vegetarian, I don't mean with lots of eggs and cheese or white flour, sugar, and fat-laden products. The latter just makes high-fat and calorie-rich, unhealthy vegetarian food. Although I would prefer a completely plant-based school meal program, if schools provided the foods described above, along with small amounts of lean animal protein (fish; lean fowl and meats; eggs, preferably free-ranged and grass-fed; and low-fat, non-sweetened yogurt—yes, leave out the cheese) this would be acceptable and beneficial as long as the meat consumption was kept to a minimum and vegetable and fruit intake was encouraged.

This also means no advertising, vending machines, or sponsorships from large food companies on school campuses that support non-whole-food items such as soft drinks, candy bars, energy drinks, and highly processed foods in general. Additionally, parents and educators alike should aim for eliminating soft drinks and caffeinated sports drinks from school cafeterias and vending machines—period! Encourage water consumption or at least mineral waters or 100 percent non-sweetened natural juices as the "in" thing, and our children will benefit immensely. Why do we allow unhealthful foods to be fed to our kids in schools as the norm? Because too many of us allow ourselves to consume this kind of diet!

A successful model that should be replicated across the country for healthy nutrition advocacy for school children, as well as educating the public and policy makers on the importance of whole-food, plant-based school nutrition, is the New York Coalition for Healthy School Foods (Healthyschoolfood.org). This group helped create the excellent illustration shown at the end of Chapter, 1 "U.S. Food Consumption as a % of Calories" for which I am very thankful, since it makes teaching about the problems of U.S. food consumption patterns simple and evident.

Diet and the Big Three:
School Behavior, Criminality, and Work Productivity

Another wonderful interview I had the privilege of conducting was with Barbara Stitt, former chief probation officer in Ohio for two decades; former co-owner of the whole-food bakery Natural Ovens; and book author, speaker, and child nutrition advocate. This interview was profound in three ways. First, she discovered that feeding probationers whole-food, unrefined diets reduced their recidivism from getting into trouble again from 85 percent down to 15 percent. Second, she and her husband, Paul Stitt, fed their more than 120 employees daily at their Natural Ovens bakery only whole foods, resulting in marked reductions in healthcare claims, increased work productivity in their employees, and general enhanced employee contentment. Third, she and her husband showed that you can go into a problem school (in this case an alternative high school in Appleton, Wisconsin), serve only whole food in their cafeteria, and turn around the students' behavior. This school's turnaround was known as the "Miracle in Wisconsin." This school was featured in the movie *Supersize Me* as a nutrition success story.

So much good would occur if Paul and Barbara's professional examples of incorporating simple whole-food nutrition were duplicated by other American businesses, schools, and governmental agencies.[54]

Finally, children must get back to being physically active. Playing outside shouldn't be a novel idea! Physical education has to be strongly encouraged, if not mandatory, even if it is just a walking class. And though it likely goes without saying, controlling the hours a child sits behind a computer screen or in front of a television is critical. That's on you, parents!

Are You Beginning to See the Picture?

It is so obvious why we are sick and chronically ill in this country (and the world). It doesn't take a rocket scientist to figure it out. Just stop and think—and *look around you!* The next time you go to a restaurant, just look at the people and what they eat. Do it at your next family gathering, at the grocery store, or at work. It's not being judgmental. It's using your brain and your common sense. We have to stop thinking that "normal" is being overweight, stuffed after a meal, or taking multiple medications starting at the age of forty. It's not!

Why do we think that three days per week of twenty minutes of exercise is something impressive when for millennia we foraged hours per day for food? Why do we allow highly processed foods to be the norm of our diet when for millions of years we ate whole, non-processed foods? Simple causes, simple solutions. We don't have to spend another dime of research to fix our healthcare crisis!

Real Prevention Is the Only Answer

Our present-day disease care model is doomed to failure. As former U.S. President Bill Clinton told Sanjay Gupta, MD, during his March 2009 interview on *Larry King Live*, no matter what type of plan we put in place to cover everyone with insurance or reduce inefficiencies in the system itself, without incorporating *disease prevention* into our lifestyles, we will fail at real healthcare reform. We will fail because the number of people with chronic disease will keep growing and any new healthcare package will simply cover more unhealthy people with chronic diseases, not create fewer of them. The percentage of our gross national product (GNP) spent on healthcare will continue to rise (presently 16.5 percent—highest in the world) to 18 or 19 percent of our GNP, and we will not be able to afford this disease-oriented healthcare system.[55]

I heard President Obama, in a television statement, say essentially the same thing. If we don't get healthcare expenses under control, not just by being more efficient but by *prevention*, in the next decade or two, healthcare expenditures could go to 20 percent of our GNP, or one-fifth of what our nation produces. If you read *President Obama's Fiscal 2010 Budget: Transforming and Modernizing America's Health Care System* from the Office of Budget and Management, it emphasizes prevention, which is good, but I think this following statement is grossly understated: "Over a third of all illness is the result of poor diet, lack of exercise, and smoking. Indeed, obesity alone leads to many expensive, chronic conditions including high blood pressure, heart disease, diabetes, and even cancer."[56]

According to our own Centers for Disease Control and Prevention (CDC), 70 percent of U.S. deaths come from chronic disease. These highly preventable chronic diseases account for 75 percent of our healthcare expenditures. The CDC states that the major risk factors for these chronic diseases are lack of physical activity, poor nutrition, tobacco use, and excessive alcohol consumption.[57]

The WHO states that chronic diseases are responsible for 60 percent of all deaths worldwide, and if the major risk factors for chronic disease were eliminated—lack of physical activity, poor nutrition, and tobacco use—at least 80 percent of heart disease, stroke, and type 2 diabetes would be prevented and 40 percent of cancers.[58]

Those are incredibly powerful statements emphasizing that preventing chronic disease with basic lifestyle changes should be the crux of any healthcare reform package. So don't blame the government! Real healthcare reform is not a political solution. It's you looking in the mirror, taking the information from this book and others, and changing your lifestyle so you dramatically reduce your chronic disease risk and stay away from the medical-industrial complex. There is no healthcare reform that will do more for you than getting off your behind and exercising and putting whole unprocessed food into your mouth. Period!

This is why I say staying healthy and living lifestyle programs such as the **TRIAD Wellness Program** of diet, exercise, and positive mental conditioning are patriotic. An act of patriotism in the twenty-first century is eating good food, getting exercise, reducing your weight, and preventing chronic disease. Even if we could afford these skyrocketing expenditures, what is our workforce going to look like? What is their productivity going to be like when competing on the world stage? Not good!

If we the people follow the *9 Simple Steps to Optimal Health,* then we will be amazed at the health and vitality we will be able to achieve in a very short time at a fraction of the cost compared to what we are spending for our healthcare dollar.

In an interview I conducted with Dr. T. Colin Campbell, co-author of the book *The China Study* and co-investigator of the famous China Project, he said something quite profound (and something I believe):

> "...I suggest that 80 to 90 percent at least of the diseases we now have in our society is really attributed to diet and to the fact that we have strayed from what really is the most natural and healthiest way to eat: Namely consuming a whole plant-based food (diet)."[59]

I hope by now you understand **what** the problem of *chronic diseases* is, **where** chronic diseases come from, and **who** they affect. My guess is that you now have a good idea of **how** to prevent these conditions and achieve good health. Let's go do it!

Chapter 6

Expect Good Health!

By this point, I hope you can see that the problems of poor health and chronic disease are basic—and so are the solutions. If I've done my job, then you have a general understanding of how we got here, what the problems are, and the solutions to the problems (diet, exercise, mental conditioning). What I think you may not have are the simple awareness, tools, and the *belief* that you can incorporate these actions into your busy life and get results. I know you can! I have seen patients do it and have experienced it myself. And as my beloved mother would say as she huffed and puffed across my dance floor with her oxygen line attached and her walker moving noisily, "*You can do it!*" Let's get started!

Make Your Health a Fun Part-Time Job

One way or another, you are eventually going to have to spend time on your health. Many people, once they reach their fifties, visit their doctor's office on a regular basis for some chronic complaint. Some even wind up in the back of an ambulance or in a hospital bed. You could resign yourself to this kind of aging process—or you could go to the gym regularly, take daily walks, and spend a little extra time shopping for and preparing healthy food. The choice is yours. How would you rather spend your time?

It takes hardly any extra time to walk up stairs versus taking an escalator. It takes the same amount of time to push your shopping cart around the grocery store picking out fruit, vegetables, beans, nuts, seeds, and whole grains as it does to get ice cream, white bread, fatty meats, and pastries. It may even take less time to walk across the parking lot instead of driving around for five or ten minutes finding the closest parking space. Yes, you have the time! Don't tell me—or, more importantly, you—that you don't have time! You'll find the time to go to the doctor's visit, go to the hospital, or get some lab tests done if you have to. If you are thinking and aware, you can add a phenomenal amount of health-promoting activities into your normal, daily routine. I know you can!

So Where Is the "Fun Part?"

The key to staying healthy and being healthy is doing things as part of your lifestyle that are fun and that help maintain your health. My brother has ridden his bicycle to work for more than thirty years. Over the years, that ride has taken anywhere from probably five minutes to an hour or so each way. So he rides to work as a necessity, but he also likes to ride his bicycle. In addition, my brother likes to coach soccer (via four girls over the years) and he referees soccer as well. While he enjoys refereeing soccer, he is also running up and down a field for a couple of hours each game getting solid exercise. My brother also teaches wilderness photography, so for "work" he takes people on beautiful scenic hikes to Yosemite. These are all perfect examples of making your health a fun part-time job!

Of course, you can also incorporate your healthy activities into your leisure time. For example, I am a swing and salsa dancer. These have become major forms of movement and aerobic exercise for me, with a little running, stair-stepper, and elliptical rider thrown on top. Dancing really makes your health a fun part-time job! I am around friends, I am listening to great music, it is convenient for me because it fits into my busy lifestyle, and I love to partner dance. But here is a little "pearl of wisdom": A lot of people think I am a bit crazy and have too much energy, because when I come to dance I dance straight for an hour or two. I don't stop for too long. There is a reason: Dance can be very aerobic or mildly aerobic, depending on how you do it and the type of dance you do.

If you stand around and dance one out of every three or four songs, you are "wasting" 50 to 75 percent of the time that could be spent moving to improve or maintain your health.

That is why I try to dance constantly for the time I have to dance, and I add a little extra aerobics to keep up my cardiovascular health. I am always thinking about how to make an activity really benefit my health while at the same time enjoying it. I only have so much time. I might dance thirty to forty dances in a two-hour period, whereas someone else might dance five or ten times in that same two-hour period. I don't have time to waste!

I have also learned to enjoy eating healthy food. While I am not a purist, it's enjoyable and fun for me to eat an unprocessed, whole-food, plant-rich diet. It can be just as fun to learn how to be creative and cook delicious, wholesome foods as it is to cook high-calorie and processed foods. The same goes for eating out. Good, healthy food can be found just about anywhere.

The Bottom Line: Enjoy Your Healthy Lifestyle

We all have to spend time attending to our health. If you can build a healthy lifestyle that you enjoy, then you are many giant steps ahead of those whose time commitment to their health is spent in suffering and frustration.

Simple health habits, when part of your "fun" lifestyle, practiced daily and consistently, will provide you with incredible health in the long run. Would you rather live life to the fullest or stop doing things you love in order to go visit the doctor and spend extra money on medication, office visits, tests, and procedures that are anything but pleasant? *I don't care if your health insurance or the government pays for your visits, medications, or procedures 100 percent! It's still not fun to spend the time and energy doing these things, not to mention not feeling well.* Either way, taking care of your health is eventually going to become a part-time job. It's up to you whether you want it to be fun and life-enhancing or miserable and all about inconvenience and suffering. If you choose fun—and I bet you will—then keep reading and I will show you how.

Have a *Staying Healthy* Mentality

Recently, a mid-fifty-year-old buddy of mine was trying to get new health insurance for his wife and himself. While shopping around, one of the insurance reps asked him how many medications he and his wife were on. When he said none she was surprised—so surprised that she repeated the question. The insurance representative said it's very rare for a mid-fifty-year-old adult in the United States trying to get health insurance to be free of taking multiple medications. That is mind-blowing. Our expectations as a society are upside down. I am not against medications when absolutely needed, but my goal is to keep people off them. My normal expectation for a fifty-year-old is to be on *no medication*! A few daily supplements, yes. Medications, no! I don't want to sound like a hypocrite. I'll take a Tylenol for a headache or an antibiotic for a real infection, but I don't picture myself being on any chronic medication—ever! It could happen, but I don't picture it no matter how old I get, and I try to live like I won't.

We have to shift our thinking. If you go to a physician's office with the expectation of getting fixed by a medication or vitamin supplement, you are missing the boat. You should be going to a health professional mostly for coaching, teaching, reassurance, and maybe an occasional short-term medication(s) with the intention of getting off of it.

I find this attitude working in integrative or complementary medicine practices as well. You can have a "fix me" and "medication" mentality when seeking alternative approaches. Same rules apply: Don't expect your supplements or the alternative modality to magically "leapfrog" the need to get off your butt and move your body daily, eat whole foods, get leaner, get some sleep, deal with relationships, etc. It's not going to happen. While supplements are inherently much safer than pharmaceuticals and ideally work to "normalize" body biochemistry, the "fix me" mentality still permeates much too much in those who seek alternative approaches as well.

With that said about our "take a pill" and "fix me" mentality, let's talk a moment about one of the ten leading causes of death in the United States—adverse drug reactions (ADRs).

Drugs Reactions: A Leading Cause of Death

What people don't realize in our "pill-popping" culture is that ADRs are one of the top ten leading causes of death in this country, at over a hundred thousand deaths annually (and this figure was for hospitalized patients only).[1] Use pharmaceuticals correctly and get off them! Always have the mentality when you go to your doctor's office to ask, "What do I have to do, change, or achieve to get off this medicine(s)?" If you don't ask or have that mentality, it's much easier for your health practitioner to just check off that you're taking the medication right and not having any obvious side effects. Doctors don't usually ask you, "Do you want to get off your chronic medication?"

In a traditional doctor's defense, doctors have no time to spend with a patient to really look at the whole person. They have very little, if any, experience seeing food manipulation in a patient really changing people dramatically, and they are not studying, as their main focus, foods and how to apply nutritional biochemistry to solve problems. They are thinking medication because that's who "reps" their offices, that's who funds their educational symposiums, and that's how they were trained—in a disease care model that treats acute and chronic symptoms with medications. *You* have to ask your practitioner, "No, seriously, Dr. Smith. I want to get off these medications. How do I do it? *What do I have to do with my lifestyle to get this done?* What do I have to change?" It will be interesting to see what answers you get. Let me know!

Medications and Chronic Disease

Virtually all the pharmaceuticals for the chronic diseases I have been talking about treat the symptoms of the disease, not the disease process itself. They don't cure! So if you do nothing, you're on these medications, and probably more and more medications, for the rest of your life. Continue to do nothing and you are going to get more pills and probably more side effects. Some of them might be life threatening, especially with more combinations of medications.

I have no doubt that, when you have a long list of medications, some of the newer medications are given to you to treat some of the side effects of the older medications, not to mention the nutritional deficiencies that many of these medications cause. Remember that someone has to fulfill the statistics of ADRs being among the top ten leading causes of death in the United States. Don't let it be you! Have the mentality of changing your lifestyle so you can get off the medications.

Normal Is Being Healthy, Not Being Sick

Americans in general are so used to seeing unhealthy people they think being unhealthy with the chronic diseases mentioned previously is normal. It is not! The normal human condition is to be fit, lean, energetic, and active.

When you read about healthy aging "Blue Zone" cultures like the Okinawan centenarians, Nicoyans in Costa Rica, Sardinians in Italy, and Ikarians in Greece, they don't have concepts of rest homes and chronic disease. They envision themselves using a machete at one hundred to cut the grass, teach karate at ninety-plus years of age, ride a bicycle up and down hills, or herd their sheep into their eighties.

We really need to grasp and visualize that the "normal" state of humans is not being sick, being on multiple medications, and visiting doctors frequently. It's just the opposite. If you don't have this vision of health, it isn't going to happen. Visualize your optimal state of health daily, which just happens to be the ninth *Simple Step to Optimal Health!*

There are three easy to read books that I highly recommend on healthy living and aging that should be *must reads* for all Americans to create real healthcare reform and vibrant health: *The Blue Zone* (2008), *The Okinawa Program* (2001), and *Healthy at 100* (2007).

Chapter 7
STAYING HEALTHY PRINCIPLES

The Wheel of Health

Your health is like a bicycle tire. You have a bunch of loose spokes and your wheel (health and wellness) is going "the-thump-the-thump-the-thump." Not a smooth ride! You have been told by one bike mechanic (doctor) that it is one spoke, and when he or she just focuses on that one spoke, you might get a little bit of temporary improvement. You see another bike mechanic, and he says it's another spoke that's the problem. He just focuses on that one. Same thing: a little improvement, but it's not enough. You go to another mechanic, and he says, "Hell, let's get rid of the whole darn tire (body part) and just get a new one!"

This is how some health professionals have been looking at your health. Why? They were trained not to look at the whole tire or fix multiple spokes. More importantly, physicians are reimbursed not for keeping all the spokes tightened and moving smoothly, but for fixing one individual broken spoke that they know a lot about. *They also have no economic incentive* to maintain the other spokes, tire, wheel bearings, air in the tires, and on and on—even though that spoke is going to continue to break because the rest of the wheel is ignored. They get their economic reward for all their time and education for fixing the broken spoke.

We have a lot of brilliant spoke fixers in the United States, many of them much smarter than I am, but—are you catching my train of thought? This is a critically important concept if we are to fix our healthcare system. The economic incentives in the past (and now) for health professionals is to wait for disease to happen, then jump in and fix it—just the part that is broken and not the multiple pathways (spokes) that led to the broken part.

For a fracture or torn cartilage, this type of medicine is needed and appreciated. For chronic diseases (heart disease, diabetes, cancers, bone loss, etc.), there is some initial benefit, but in the long run, because you are only dealing with the spoke and not the whole wheel of why this chronic disease exists, it is bound to fail therapeutically, economically, and for the individual and society.

I look at your health this way: You come to me with a variety of complaints and a few major ones. I look at these complaints as the endpoint of a group of loose spokes. Some I will be able to identify; some I won't. Maybe I can't help you tighten all the loose spokes, but if I help you tighten four or five spokes at once, then your wheel (wellness) begins to turn a bit better. With time, if we do things right and keep tightening four or five of these spokes (or a few more that we discover), your wheel begins to "self-tighten" its own spokes, and your wheel of health begins to really turn smoothly. You begin to cruise with your health. Then we just keep gently tightening the majority of the spokes with good lifestyle (i.e., **TRIAD Wellness Program**) and you ride smoothly through life.

Why Traditional Medicine Fails

Traditional medicine has specialties for each individual spoke in your wheel of health. There is nothing wrong with that if you "bust" that spoke. When I needed both my ACLs repaired, I wanted the orthopedic knee specialist whose expertise was ACL reconstruction to do the job.

Yes, we need specialists—but we should be in a position to need a lot *fewer* of them. As long as the vast majority of reimbursement in our medical care model goes to those who fix the "busted spokes" (i.e., heart surgeries, angioplasties, hip and knee replacements, cataract surgeries, etc.) and not to those who help the public keep the daily self-tightening of their major spokes in check (hopefully primary care physicians and other allied health professionals), then we are going to have more and more people with more and more busted spokes, which are more costly to fix and result in a lot more disability.

It is true that our ever-evolving medical technology advances impressively over time, but the overall functional health of our society doesn't improve because we are doing too little to prevent these spokes from going bad in the first place. Sooner or later individuals, health insurance companies, and governments will no longer be able to pay for these repairs, and we will go bankrupt or just not take care of certain groups of people. This is the direction and present state of U.S. healthcare in which we find ourselves today.

I would like to make a very important point about the meaning of "preventive medicine." When I say preventive medicine, I'm not talking about a government program making children and adults get more and more vaccinations or pap smears and mammograms. I'm talking about economic incentives that teach, encourage, and demand that people eat right, get exercise, lose weight, and prevent and reverse the chronic diseases I have been talking about.

How Alternative Medicine May Fail

There is no magic bullet to being healthy. Good health is a daily consistent practice of simple principles and disciplines that incorporate physical activity; a whole-food, unprocessed, vegetable-based diet; and a positive, loving mental outlook on life. Any practice that improves one, two, or all three of these areas is going to improve the overall health of the individual and society.

Alternative medicine will fail if it puts more emphasis on so-called natural therapies than on the person's lifestyle of regular disciplines that enhance the synergy of diet, exercise, and mind-body practices in addition to these natural therapies.

I have been around a few famous health gurus since 1983 when I started practicing integrative and primary care medicine. A good number don't appear to practice what they preach and don't look all that healthy. All I can say is that alternative practitioners better provide the basics of creating a wellness lifestyle, then add on less-invasive, science-based natural therapies. The industry can't get wrapped up in money-making products or modalities, or we are just the same as the pharmaceutical industry, pushing to sell more products to treat disease instead of preventing disease. *The emphasis has to be on prevention by living healthy lifestyles, not by depending on new, amazing natural products.* That is what the **TRIAD Wellness Program** is about.

Busting the "Spoke Busters": The TRIAD Wellness Program

The integration of what kind of fuel we ingest (diet), how we move our bodies (exercise), and how we think about our lives and health (mind-body) makes up the essence of the **TRIAD Wellness Program** approach and the *9 Simple Steps to Optimal Health* I have mentioned. The goal is to tighten the basic spokes gently but consistently every day of our lives so that our wheel of health turns smoothly. Or, if we get a busted spoke, we repair it quickly, and since the other spokes are all in check, we get well faster and with less expense and loss of function and pain.

Truly healthy aging populations naturally live the **TRIAD Wellness** approach:

- They eat whole, unprocessed foods that are available to them, they eat lots of unrefined, fresh plant foods, and they don't consume excess calories.
- Animal foods are generally used sparingly in addition to indigenous plant foods. They are not the main part of the diet.
- They practice under-eating (diet).
- They move every day using a mixture of aerobic-type movement along with natural strength and flexibility exercise (exercise). We would call it "cross-training."
- They have a deep sense and vision of their daily purpose and their place in the universe, and they roll with life's ups and downs (mind-body). They have strong social bonds.

The unique design of the **TRIAD Wellness Program** is to incorporate these three phases into the lives of people like you and me in this busy, modern world.

The Body: Falling Apart or Always Healing?

We are all aging, and our physical body will die someday, so I guess you could say that we are always falling apart. That is not the way I choose to believe and feel about how my body works. I believe your body is always trying to come back to balance—always trying to heal itself. If I just get out of the way and give it what it needs—real whole food, physical activity, sunshine, a clean environment, good sleep, challenges but not overwhelming stress, and clear visions of what my true passions are (*9 Simple Steps*)—it will perform beautifully until I am 110! This age just popped into my head in the last several years. As I see it, I am not quite halfway through my life yet! My body wants to be well. It is programmed to be well, and so is yours. Just give it what it needs and as little as possible of what it doesn't need, and it will do the rest magnificently. Believe it!

Chapter 8

THE FOUNDATION FOR A *STAYING HEALTHY* DIET

The "D" word—diet—doesn't often excite people. This chapter will give you a clearer understanding of where our diet may have come from, examines some common components to many popular diet programs, and then gives some basic rules about what to eat, how to shop, and what to have in your house.

Where Did the Human Diet Come From?

Our primate ancestors were predominantly tree dwellers who consumed what is called the "simian diet," which consisted mainly of leaves, fruit, nuts, and things that they could gather from being tree dwellers.[1] They didn't consume animal products aside from maybe a few bugs, worms, and things with all the vegetation they consumed.

When this population exceeded the space or area that was available in the tree world, they came down on the ground and started to eat leaves, roots, fruit, nuts, and then eventually flesh food—first "leftovers" or carrion (dead animal carcass), and then man learned with the proper tools how to hunt and kill his own food. This is commonly called the Paleolithic diet, hunter-gatherer or caveman type of diet, which occurred possibly from 2.5 million years ago to 10,000 years ago.[2] Modern day hunter-gatherers have been estimated to obtain more than 50 percent of their daily energy intake from animal foods. Most of their food calories come from wild animal products, vegetables, fruits, and nuts.[3]

Since considerable grain consumption and production is only about ten thousand years old, some say that grains are not optimal to eat because we couldn't have evolved that fast from our hunter-gatherer, or Paleolithic, roots.

Indigenous diets are created from a group of people over hundreds or even thousands of years using their traditional knowledge to make a complete diet of local foods.[4] An indigenous diet could be a hunter-gather type diet or a diet that has evolved over hundreds of years in a particular location, like in some of the Blue Zone areas of the world: Okinawa (Japan), Sardinia (Italy), Nicoya (Costa Rica), Hunza (Pakistan), or Ikaria (Greece). Today's modern indigenous diets have traditional people eating local and fresh foods that are in season. If an indigenous population lives near a river or ocean, they might consume fish, local vegetation, fruit, and some form of unrefined starchy foods. If they live inland, they may be more vegetarian, with some grain, starchy vegetables, and root crops; or they may eat hunted game or free-ranged domestic animals with the same whole-food vegetarian base.

One key component when healthy indigenous cultures eat animal products is that they are usually free-ranged or wild animals. Instead of the animals consuming feedlot grains and beans and other things (hormones and antibiotics), the animals feed on local, usually green, vegetation that has a better fatty acid profile than feedlot food. In other words, domesticated free-range-fed animals (or wild animals) should have a more anti-inflammatory fatty acid profile compared to our mass-raised and mass-slaughtered feedlot animals. Wild and free-range animals are generally more lean and not as fatty as factory-farmed animals. Also, the quantity of meat that modern indigenous cultures eat is generally less than what present day urbanized societies consume.[5]

There is a lot of debate about what our natural diet should be (and there isn't going to be agreement anytime soon). You can go on the Internet and see the polarity of beliefs on what the best diet is. Instead of looking at the differences, let's look at what is common to many of the diets, and then let's look at what the people who live the longest eat in order to come up with some basic guidelines. Then, I hope, it won't be so confusing. Because it really isn't!

Animal vs. Plant Foods in the Human Diet

Dr. Marion Nestle, a well-respected nutrition expert and author of three books (*Food Politics,* 2002; *Safe Food,* 2003; and *What To Eat,* 2006) writes on the issue of the Paleolithic diet of meat (animal products), vegetables, fruit and nuts (but generally grain free) and compares it to the modern need for a more plant-based diet. According to her research:

> "...As economies changed from scarcity to abundance, principal diet-related diseases have shifted from nutrient deficiencies to chronic diseases related to dietary excesses. This shift has led to increasing scientific consensus that eating more plant foods but fewer animal foods would best promote health. This consensus is based on research relating dietary factors to chronic disease risks and to observations of exceptionally low chronic disease rates among people consuming vegetarian, Mediterranean, and Asian diets. One challenge to this consensus is the idea that Paleolithic man consumed more meat than currently recommended, and that this pattern is genetically determined. If such exists, a genetic basis for ideal proportions of plant or animal foods is difficult to determine; hominoid primates are largely vegetarian, current hunter-gatherer groups rely on foods that can be obtained most conveniently, and the archeological record is insufficient to determine whether plants or animals predominated. Most evidence suggests that a shift to largely plant-based diets would reduce chronic disease risks among industrialized and rapidly industrializing populations. To accomplish this shift, it will be necessary to overcome marketplace barriers and to develop new policies that will encourage greater consumption of fruit, vegetables, and grains as a means to promote public health."[6]

According to Dr. Loren Cordain (and Dr. James H O'Keefe), one of the premier researchers and proponents of the Paleolithic diet and author of *The Paleo Diet* (2002) and *The Paleo Diet For Athletes* (2005):

"Man's ancestors foraged or hunted for wild plants and animals in their natural world. When hunter-gatherer societies transitioned to an agricultural grain-based diet, their general health deteriorated. Those who switched to grain-based diets had shorter life spans, higher childhood mortality, and a higher incidence of osteoporosis, rickets, and other vitamin/mineral deficiencies....The Paleolithic diet compared with the average modern American diet contained 2 to 3 times more fiber, 1.5 to 2.0 times more polyunsaturated and monounsaturated fats, 4 times more omega-3 fats, and 60–70% less saturated fat. Protein intake was 2 to 3 times higher, and potassium intake was 3 to 4 times higher, while sodium intake was 4 to 5 times lower. The Paleolithic diet contained no refined grains and sugars except for honey. In the growing season, an abundance of fruits, berries, and vegetables were consumed.

"...The hunter-gatherer diet was high in beneficial phyto-chemicals and antioxidants...Omega-3 fats were abundant in the Paleolithic diet. The small amount of fat in algae, grasses, and leaves is rich in omega-3 fatty acids, which become more concentrated in larger animals up through both land and ma-rine food chains, especially in fish and larger grazing animals... Monounsaturated fats made up half of the total fat in the diets of hunter-gatherers. Monounsaturated fats have been shown to be cardioprotective. Hunter-gatherers consumed nuts as sources of calorie-dense, highly nutritious foods that were often available in non-summer months. Typically, nuts are 80% fat, and most of this is from monounsaturated and polyunsaturated fats, includ-ing some omega-3 fats...Paleolithic humans lived in temperate climates where, during the winter months, plant food was not available. Early humans adapted to these conditions by consum-ing meat, organs, marrow, and fat from animals during the win-ter months. These meat-based hunter-gatherer diets were non-atherogenic. The flesh of wild game is about 2-4% fat and has relatively high amounts of monounsaturated fats and omega-3 fats compared with the flesh of fatty grain-produced domestic animals, which contains 20-25% fat, much of which is in the form of saturated fat...

"...The hunter-gatherers were very physically active, walking and running 5–10 miles a day to forage for food and hunted food sources. They cross-trained by lifting, carrying, climbing, stretching, leaping, and whatever else was necessary to secure food and protect themselves. They also had recovery days. Man's Paleolithic ancestors did aerobic training, resistance training, and flexibility exercises."[7] (From O'Keefe JH Jr, Cordain L. *Cardiovascular disease resulting from a diet and lifestyle at odds with our paleolithic genome: how to become a 21st-century hunter-gatherer.* Mayo Clin Proc. 2004; 79(1):101–108. Used with permission.)

What Does This Mean for Us Today?

Unfortunately, we will never know how long Paleolithic man would have lived with his diet and lifestyle in our modern, urbanized society to compare its benefits with what we know today, especially in a rapidly aging world. Though the dwindling hunter-gatherer populations of today may have low incidences of chronic diseases with their higher animal foods yet generally grain-free diets, the diets of the longest living people in the world include some grains. For example, rice and noodles in the Okinawans, wheat bread in the Sardinians, and multiple grains in the Seventh Day Adventists. Most all other healthy aging or Blue Zone populations have a staple grain or grains.

We also know that we no longer live the way humans did in the Paleolithic world. The types of meats commonly available to the masses are not lean, hunted wild game rich in omega-3 fatty acids and low in total fat. Yes, there is grass-fed, free-ranged animals for those who have access and who can afford these animal products. Yet I have never received a good answer from anyone where all this "free-range" land is going to come from to raise these types of animals to feed the ever-increasing world population's appetite for animal foods.

Furthermore, the average urbanized citizen isn't foraging and "cross-training" for food five to ten miles per day or walking six or so hours per day over difficult terrain (well, maybe a Sardinian goat/sheep herder is!). Therefore, we don't need as much of the calorie-dense food that can come from animals, especially mass-produced, factory-farmed animals.

The Okinawan elders are probably the best-studied and documented group of centenarians (hundred-year-olds) in the world.[8] Thanks to the detailed and efficient Japanese government, excellent family registries (*koseki*) on birth dates have been kept since 1879, allowing for true age confirmation of these centenarians. The Japanese government sponsored the Okinawa Centenarian Study established in 1976, which looked at diseases; risk factors; biochemical parameters, including hormones and diet; lifestyle; and social structure in this exceptional group of people. Combining this data with current data on aging, nutrition, and prevention provides an excellent model for creating healthy and functionally aging societies. *The Okinawa Program* (2001) is one of the great health books of all time (as is *The Okinawa Diet Plan,* 2005). These books really are a blueprint for real healthcare reform since they document so many parameters of healthful and functional longevity in the modern world.

The Okinawans are even more remarkable as a population that can teach us how to live healthfully because in present-day Okinawa, there is a striking dichotomy in health and longevity between the elders and their children and grandchildren. The Okinawan elders still eat much of their traditional diet high in plant foods, moderate amounts of fish, and smaller amounts of meat. Their diet is rich in vegetables and soy foods, grains, beans, small amounts of fruit, and minimal dairy products. The elders remain functionally healthy into their eighties, nineties, and one hundreds. On the other hand, the younger generations of Okinawans in the same geographic locations with the same genes are experiencing dramatic increases in obesity, diabetes, and cardiovascular diseases that can be directly traced to their consumption of highly processed and fast foods as a direct result of Western influence in the area. This division of health is made so blatantly evident in a YouTube video by Dr. Sanjay Gupta of CNN entitled, "Western Diet: A Killer in Okinawa. Part II."[9] I send this short clip to all my patients trying to get the point across that good health is mostly lifestyle and not our genes. The sad part is that the Okinawan elders are dying out, and the younger Okinawan generations adopting the Western diet are dying young—many times before their long-living parents.

Diet of Okinawan Elders vs. American Diet

Meat, poultry, eggs	3%	29%
Calcium-rich foods	2% (dairy, seaweed)	23% (dairy)
Vegetables	34%	16%
Fruit	6%	20%
Flavonoid foods (soy)	12%	< 1%
Grains	32%	11%
Omega 3 foods	11% (fish)	< 1% (fish)

Note: Percentages by weight of a particular food.
Source: Bradley J. Willcox, MD; D. Craig Willcox, PhD; and Makoto Suzuki, MD, PhD.
The Okinawa Program: How the World's Longest-Lived People Achieve Everlasting Health—And How You Can Too. (New York: Three Rivers Press, 2001), 71.

Each successful aging culture, in its geographic location, has foods that are high in antioxidant properties and rich in beneficial phytonutrients. For example, the Okinawans used to eat a lot of imo or sweet potato; it was the only thing that would grow during some very harsh times. As it turns out, imo has an excellent glycemic response (slow blood sugar absorption) and is very high in beta-carotene. They drink lots of green tea with protective catechins. They eat lots of antioxidant rich vegetables and a high quantity of soy products rich in isoflavones.[10] The long living Sardinians in Italy might use more tomato products containing lycopene, fava beans rich in protein and fiber, milk and cheese containing the anti-inflammatory substance arzanol from goats grazing on the dwarf curry plant, or resveratrol in their homemade red wine.[11] Both cultures are getting powerful antioxidants and phytochemicals from their "local" foods that provide protection against chronic disease.

The key is that these "super" foods are usually, though not always, plant foods—especially vegetables and fruit. That's where the magic is: in the plants (or some animal products that eat the protective plant compounds). Also, it is the unique compound surrounded by known and unknown synergistic plant compounds, not the isolated substance, that creates the enhanced health benefits. That means that eating the whole food is far and away more effective than simply popping a supplement extracted from some exotic super-food. The take-home point: a healthy diet is comprised of a variety of unrefined, local plant and vegetable foods and may or may not contain small amounts of animal foods.

The Importance of Studying Modern Day Blue Zone Cultures

While I think it is interesting and educational to study the different dietary patterns from which we evolved (Simian, Paleolithic, Neolithic), I think it is considerably more important and urgent to study modern-day healthy aging population's (Blue Zone) dietary (and lifestyle) patterns. These modern-day cultures have the same genetics as our evolutionary ancestors, but because they are living relatively free from chronic diseases and remain highly functional into their eighties, nineties, and one hundreds, the environment with which they "bathe" their genes—which includes the foods they eat, the physical activity they get, and their social interactions and mind-set—are critically important to learn from so we can solve our current healthcare crisis. If we wipe out chronic diseases, or delay them significantly, like many of these healthy aging cultures do, then we are going to go a long way in solving the U.S. and the world's healthcare crisis.

Remember, 75 percent of the U.S. healthcare budget goes to treat chronic disease. We should be studying urgently these healthy aging populations in the U.S. and abroad, and keeping track of their diet, lifestyle, and biochemical data on what is optimal and set programs up to emulate some of these principles in the modern world.[12] This why I frequently reference these populations throughout this book. They are living laboratories that can give us simple, doable solutions to our healthcare crisis. We need to study them before these populations die out. As mentioned in Chapter 6, my favorite books on this subject are *The Blue Zone* (2008), *The Okinawa Program* (2001), *The Okinawa Diet Plan* (2004), and *Healthy at 100* (2007).

"One-Rule Diet"

If I had to make a "one-rule diet," it would be simply to eat whole, unprocessed food. That's it! This by itself would wipe out a large portion of chronic diseases—your grocery store would probably be a fraction of its size if only whole, unprocessed foods were available (fruit, vegetables, beans, whole grains, nuts, seeds, eggs, fish, poultry, and meat; dairy products are not whole foods, in my opinion). Even if you did the opposite of what I recommend with regard to portions of food groups (more than half your food intake as vegetables and more than 90 percent plant foods), but still ate only whole unprocessed foods, the average American would do considerably better. This is because we would not be eating refined grains, added fats and oils, added calorie sweeteners, creams and cheeses, or other calorie-dense, nutrient-poor foods. This one rule leaves only one of the unhealthy dietary changes that have occurred over the last century resulting in excess calories to be present: the increased consumption of predominantly factory-farmed meats.

Then Why No Meat?

Though I would prefer everyone be vegans, the data is undeniable that you can consume animal products and be healthy. The living data clearly show that people can eat animal foods with significant amounts of unrefined plant foods and live long and healthy lives. We cannot, however, simply analyze this data in a vacuum. Rather we must look at the global big picture and ask ourselves three questions:

First, would it be possible to make some universal diet changes that will *quickly* and *dramatically* improve the overall health and environment of people all over the world? The answer to this question is a resounding yes! An unrefined, high micronutrient-dense plant-based diet would do this.

Second, can the world's resources and environment support close to 7 billion-plus people eating animal foods as we currently do in the West or developed countries, or as current hunter-gatherer populations consuming a Paleolithic-like diet? The answer is a resounding *no it can't!*

Even if health-minded meat eaters tried to eat free-ranged, antibiotic-free, and hormone-free animal foods (or hunted game), how are they going to do this for 7 billion people without destroying more precious forests or land for grazing? Where is all this open space? I frequently ask this question to my health-conscious meat-eating friends. As I previously mentioned, I have never received an answer of how. These concerns also apply to the dwindling fish stocks in the oceans and the farming of fish as a solution. If we don't learn how to intelligently and healthfully become predominantly whole food, unprocessed plant eaters, what is and will continue is factory farming of animals at an accelerated pace, with all its negatives, to feed the voracious appetite of the world's rapidly industrializing populations.

This very point about the unsustainability of animal foods consumption for the ever-growing world population was expressed by Dr. Loren Cordain, the author of the *Paleo Diet* (2002) and proponent that the Paleolithic diet is the optimal human diet. At a recent medical conference I attended (ACAM, Fall 2010), during a question and answer period Dr. Cordain was asked about the need to feed wild game or free-ranged-fed animals to school children. Dr. Cordain responded by saying that it was a shame that the optimal diet humans evolved with (Paleolithic diet) was *unsustainable* because of the ever increasing human population. He also reiterated this fact in a recent interview I did with him. These were quite interesting comments with which I concur wholeheartedly.[13]

Third, even if we could somehow sustain a healthy level of animal food consumption on a global level, would that be better for us than a whole-food, plant-based diet? It's debatable by well-intentioned and intelligent people, but personally I believe not. When was the last time you saw a study of a meat-based diet slowing or reversing heart disease, diabetes, or prostate cancer? I haven't. I am sure it's possible, but I haven't seen it. I have only seen strict plant-based studies show this.

We have an epidemic of chronic diseases worldwide that are not only causing needless human suffering but also destroying the bank accounts of countries from the direct costs of treating these chronic diseases, in addition to the loss of work productivity from unhealthy work forces. The fastest and most efficient way to reverse this trend is for the masses to consume a high micro-nutrient-dense, unprocessed, whole-food, plant-strong diet rich in vegetables, fruit, legumes, nuts and seeds, and whole grains when grains are eaten. Healthcare reform is a non-issue if we take care of business and keep ourselves healthy by preventing, delaying, and reversing chronic diseases by consuming this type of diet and we get the masses exercising.

Almost every credible health and medical organization recommends reducing animal foods intake while consuming more plant foods (although they are not willing to recommend eating only unprocessed plant foods).

A Sage's Thoughts on Modern Food Consumption

I had the privilege of interviewing Dr. David J.A. Jenkins, MD, PhD, DSc, on two separate occasions over the last two years. He is the creator of the popular *Glycemic Index* and developer of what he calls the *Dietary Portfolio,* a dietary pattern for cholesterol lowering and diabetes prevention and treatment. The *Dietary Portfolio* is a vegan diet (no animal products), with vegetables, fruit, whole grains, nuts, soy, and beans, rich in soluble and viscous fibers. This diet has not only reduced cholesterol to levels similar to the older statin drugs but has also been used to control or reverse type 2 diabetes.[14] I asked him if he had any closing comments at the end of one of his interviews. His answer was quite thought provoking. He said,

"...We've begun to realize first of all, we needed food so we (humans) got ourselves a food supply, and that's, I think, fairly secure in Western nations. Not always secure in other nations. But I think once we got a secure food supply, then we start noticing that we started developing ill health related to the security of our food supply—in other words, the abundance of our food. So I think that the third stage we are going to move into is noting that we've done terrible things to the planet in the name of a quest for food. I think we've got to start learning now to go back and correct things. We've got to start from the top downward. First of all, I think we've got to learn what foods are sustainable and still allow other species their space and their food, and their own pass-way to evolution, as it were. At the same time, we use our science to take these foods that are okay for us. They may not be as palatable and may not be as brilliant as we want, but these are the okay foods for use, and then see how we can put these back into the human diet along with physical activity and get us into a better place. But I don't think that the very egocentric way we've been approaching nutrition is appropriate because it has such a vast environmental impact. I think we've got to start looking at what we're doing to the rest of the planet, the other life forms on the planet, and start asking ourselves, is there a better way of eating? And I think if we do that and stop worrying quite as much in a focused way about how can we get more out of it ourselves, I think we'll probably end up being better overall because we will have a more complete solution to our problems if we learn how to solve the other problems we've caused other species and the rest of the planet in general."[15]

To me, the only way you can do this when approaching 7 billion people on the planet is to eat a whole-food, unprocessed, plant-based diet. Raising and eating animals for food energetically has never been a very efficient or ecologically benign process. Just think what will happen if the 1.33 billion Chinese and 1.17 billion-plus people in India continue on their "modernization" course, disre-garding their traditional plant-rich diets, and eat higher quantities of animal foods (and more added fats, oils, sugars, refined grains, etc.) as we do in the West.[16] The epidemics of heart disease, obe-sity, and other chronic diseases are going to continue to explode in those regions of the world. We, and they, will pay the price in healthcare costs and environmental destruction.

Also, I believe there is something that negatively affects our core spirit as humans by senselessly killing *billions* of animals per year for food, for really *no reason*. In the United States, we slaughter around 9 billion animals per year alone for consumption. A little bit more than 98 percent of the animals slaughtered are poultry, more than 95 percent are chicken, and less than 2 percent are red meats.[17]

I believe it is impossible for the world to be *truly* healthy and thrive as a human species on the one hand, and on the other pol-lute our environment and our bodies and senselessly kill billions of animals for food for no evolutionary or survival reason whatso-ever. There is no reason in the modern world that we have to eat animal foods to survive and thrive as a human species—none!

Diet Demystified— Common Ground of Modern Popular Diets

With so many different diets on the market, it is no wonder that people are often confused. Yet there are always common points of connection, like how the popular diets all agree on at least two things:

First, no refined carbohydrates. Some diets emphasize eating only whole grains while others might eliminate carbohydrates al-together, especially from grains. No diet that I have ever heard of encourages refined, processed carbohydrate consumption. If you think about it, and if you look at the food patterns over the last century in the United States, with the increase in refined grain con-sumption along with added fat and sweet calories, then you can see where excess carbohydrate consumption has had an adverse effect on weight. If you were only eating whole grains, beans, unprocessed starchy vegetables, and fruit, there would be a dramatic shift to better weight control. The word "carb" would not be such a bad word. In fact, "carbohydrate" is a really good word in nutrition and health. Just eat good, whole, and unprocessed carbohydrates.

Second, all diets—vegan, vegetarian, carnivore, or omnivore, low-fat or high-fat—*encourage the consumption of vegetables*. Some encourage fruit; some don't. No diet discourages vegetable consumption.

If everyone strictly adhered to the *"no refined carbohydrates"* and *"eating lots of vegetables"* components in almost all the popular diets, there would be a dramatic change in the health of our country and in other developed and developing countries. There would be a dramatic reduction in weight and excess calories, which are main causes of chronic disease. You could call this the **"Two-Rule Diet."**

So there are actually three principles that most all successful diets follow: eat unprocessed foods only, eat no refined carbohydrates, and eat lots of vegetables.

You might have observed that I keep repeating the words "unrefined," "unprocessed," and "whole." There is a reason for this. If you use these three simple words as the basis for all of your food choices, then you will dramatically change your health. **It is that simple!** You don't need a calorie counter or fifteen rules on a particular diet or excessive menus. You just need to understand what "unrefined," "unprocessed," and "whole" mean. I promised you the rules would be simple. They may not be easy initially, but they are very, very simple rules for a healthy diet.

What these rules result in if applied are the elimination of added calories to foods, an increase in protective phytochemicals, and a reduction in the glycemic response of foods resulting in lowered blood sugar and insulin levels, which reduce inflammation and risk to virtually all disease. Any dietary pattern that cuts calories, increases protective micronutrient intake, and controls blood sugar is going to do a lot of good in the modern world.

Why Eat Plant Foods?

Plant foods have everything (almost). You can live off plant foods and not eat another ounce of animal products and be absolutely and wonderfully healthy. Plant foods have protein, fat, carbohydrate, fiber, and almost all the life-preserving phytochemicals, vitamins, and minerals. If you are a strict vegan, meaning you eat no animal products, you should supplement with vitamin B12, for insurance. If you don't get adequate sunlight, you should take vitamin D. If you don't eat a lot of greens, sea vegetables, or nuts and seeds, you may need to take some omega-3 fatty acids.

When I get confused about nutrition (yes, I do at times, from all the media and Internet medical "experts"), I consider two things.

First, I tend to think of animals that are closely related to us and what they are eating. If a gorilla can be almost completely vegan (some eat termites and ants, along with whatever bugs are on the plant they are eating) and survive without consuming animal products (and dairy) for their strong muscles and bones, then so can I. A gorilla eats massive quantities of foliage and fruit—that is about it!

The second thing I do when confused is look at what healthy aging cultures eat, like the Okinawans, Sardinians, Nicoyans, Hunzas, Abhkasians, Vilcabambans, Seventh Day Adventists, Tarahumara Indians, or the cultures in the "Cold Spots" or "Blue Zones" of the world. You see very similar dietary patterns: They eat local fresh fruit and vegetables; a staple, unrefined grain (starch) usually; some beans, lentils or root vegetables; and maybe some nuts and seeds. The animal products they eat are generally more of a condiment than a big part of their plate. It may not be eaten every day, maybe only on special occasions or once or twice per week—and it is usually a free-ranged, grass-fed animal eating local vegetation (with an anti-inflammatory fat profile) and lean overall. This is a much different way of eating than the typical consumer of the Western diet.

Why Be Vegan/Vegetarian?

About fifteen or so years ago, I became a vegetarian, and around ten or more years ago, I became what I call a "sloppy" vegan. A vegetarian eats plant foods but can also, depending on the type of vegetarian, eat eggs (ovo-) or dairy products (lacto-). A vegan does not eat any animal foods. I call myself a "sloppy" vegan because I still have leather shoes, once a month or so I might have some type of dairy food or maybe something with eggs in it. I might have vegetable soup at a restaurant that might be made with chicken broth. I don't go out and buy animal foods for my home use, nor do I go out and order animal foods. I would say that I am a 99 percent-plus vegan; "sloppy" is a pretty good description! Vegetarianism is a process and evolution. Once you start, it grows on you, and aspects of it become more important to you and you continue to change.

Health and Weight Control Being a Vegetarian

Before I describe the benefits of vegetarianism on weight control, I want to make it clear that I am talking about whole-food vegetarians, eating the majority of their diet as vegetables, fruit, beans, nuts and seeds, whole grains and *minimal or no refined or processed foods.* There is nothing worse for the cause of encouraging plant-based diets than a "loud" vegetarian who is eating refined-grain products, rich in fats and added sugar; processed vegetarian foods; and virtually no vegetables and fruit—one who looks shriveled up, pale, and has to have his or her caffeine fix in order to walk. Or, a vegetarian who is overweight, eating all kinds of refined, sweet-fat-enriched flour "animal-free" foods. Please, please, my vegetarian brothers and sisters—eat whole, unrefined plant foods with tons of vegetables, fruit, beans, nuts, seeds, and moderate amounts of whole grains. (Watch for food sensitivities, especially to grains). Get some exercise and some sunlight daily. Don't be processed-food, refined-grain vegetarians or, as Dr. Cordain, the author of *The Paleo Diet,* so aptly calls these types of vegetarians, "breaditarians."[18]

Weight control is probably the biggest nemesis to worldwide health. The easy access to food (calories) makes our survival-oriented "thrifty genes" work overtime, storing excess calories as fat to protect us from when we don't have enough calories, which in modern, urbanizing life is usually never. Essentially, we were designed to store calories for periods of starvation. Thus, modern man has too many calories at his fingertips and in frequencies that we never had during our evolution.

If you want to eat a lot (like I do!) and not think about it, eat only unrefined plant foods from the following food groups, in this order: green leafy vegetables, all vegetables, fruit, beans, whole grains, and some nuts and seeds until you are lean. Then add in whole- or sprouted-grain breads. There is room for debate on the use of nuts and seeds in weight-reduction programs as part of your daily diet. There is no problem eating raw nuts or seeds in a weight-reduction program if you have some control and replace animal foods with them. Raw nuts have good fats and provide protein, fiber, and provide a degree of satiety. Also, some fat may help prevent gall bladder disease and improve vitamin absorption on a low-fat, plant based weight-reducing diet. The problem is many people eat handfuls of salted and roasted nuts (instead of raw), which have significant amounts of fat as well as salt. So I am always cautious in recommending nut and seed consumption, which are inherently very nutritious and good foods. Remember, fat has two-and-a-half times the calories of a carbohydrate or protein per gram! They are more calorie dense than a carbohydrate or protein. That's the problem. Be cautious. Maybe a quarter cup per day or less of raw nuts if on a weight loss program.

Processed foods are not good for weight control for obvious reasons: They are calorie dense from added fats and oils and calorie sweeteners (sugars) and low in fiber and beneficial nutrients because the grains are refined. Animal foods, especially factory-farmed animal foods, and dairy products are very calorie-dense foods and generally don't have beneficial fatty acid profiles and increase inflammation. They are also virtually absent of protective phytonutrients as well.

What you want to do is maintain weight without thinking about it. Your weight loss diet should be very close to your healthy lifestyle diet. To do this, you need to eat the foods with the highest nutrients per calorie (nutrient density) and the lowest amount of calories per weight (calorie density) that are packed with the most amount of protective phytonutrients (vitamins, minerals, antioxidants, phenolic compounds, etc.). This formula is found in a plant-strong diet containing lots of vegetables, fruit, beans, some whole grains, and raw nuts and seeds.

Enjoying Vegetarian Food: Is it Possible for Meat Eaters?

I am a vegetarian because of health, ecology, kindness to animals, and spiritual reasons. I didn't give up meat because I was repulsed by the taste. I loved the taste of meat! (In fact, in college I purchased a half a cow and ate steak literally every day!) If I didn't presently have in my mind the needless suffering of animals, I would periodically consume a thick porterhouse steak on the grill and then probably have a big, fat, juicy Polish sausage with sauerkraut and mustard to top off my meal. I can still taste it to this day. With that said, I don't crave meat at all. The absolute vastness of the vegan menu is awesome!

Getting over the craving for meat is easier than dairy products, caffeine, or sugar. Think of the animals, your health, or your environment. Start slowly. I allowed myself one hamburger a week, and that was the only meat I ate for several years. Then one day I read some spiritual reading and that was it. I just stopped. Vegetarianism is an evolutionary process. Just start, then it takes on a life of its own. It is a personal journey, but this journey will change you and the planet for the better.

Can You Be Strong and Be a Vegetarian?

Yes! You can be athletic and maintain excellent muscle mass if you care to as a vegan. I have maintained the same muscle mass for more than thirty years since playing college sports. Half of that time I was a meat eater and the other half I was a vegetarian, then vegan. I am as vain as any of you: I want to keep my muscles and maintain my athletic ability, too! It's easy to do on a vegan diet. Just eat a lot of whole plant foods. Nuts, seeds, and beans are concentrated sources of plant protein. Green leafy vegetables and broccoli have more protein *per calorie* than a steak.[19] Here is a list of some elite and current vegan athletes:[20]

- **Brendan Brazier**—Professional triathlete, ultra-marathon champion
- **Cat Johnson**—Professional cyclo-cross racer since 2004
- **Christine Vardaros**—Professional cycling, cyclo-cross, and road racing
- **George Laraque**—Professional hockey player
- **Mac Danzig**—Professional mixed martial artist
- **Molly Cameron**—Professional cyclo-cross racer
- **Kenneth G. Williams**—Professional vegan bodybuilder
- **Ricardo Moreira**—Professional mixed martial artist
- **Robert Cheeke**—Professional vegan bodybuilder
- **Ruth Heidrich**—Elite runner and triathlete
- **Salim Stoudamire**—Professional basketball player
- **Scott Jurek**—Professional ultra-marathoner
- **Tim VanOrden**—Profession distance runner
- **Ultramantis Black**—Professional wrestler

(Special thanks to the Colleen Holland, associate publisher of *VegNews* and its staff for their assistance in compiling this list. vegnews.com)

Tony Gonzalez, the perennial All-Pro tight end formerly of the Kansas City Chiefs and now with the Atlanta Falcons, made a dramatic switch to a vegan diet several years ago and eventually switched to a whole-food, very high plant-based diet, plus fish four times per week and free-ranged chicken a couple of times per week as his predominant animal foods.[21] He felt he needed more animal protein to maintain his large muscle mass and strength to play pro football. If you read his book, *The All-Pro Diet: Lose Fat, Build Muscle, and Live Like a Champion*, you'll see that he's eating a really clean diet that is still very highly plant-based.[22]

I hope what Tony Gonzalez has done in changing his diet to a whole-food diet and eating a lot more unprocessed, micronutrient-rich plant foods will positively influence professional athletes who are walking down a very unhealthy path, as well as non-professional athletes and kids looking at him as a role model. Instead of selling needless and potentially harmful protein supplements in gyms, they should sell Tony's book. Though it's not a vegan diet, it gets people pointed in the plant-strong direction.

It should also be noted that Tony Gonzalez was significantly influenced to change to a more unprocessed plant-based diet after reading *The China Study* by T. Colin Campbell, PhD, which provides the science and evidence behind a worldwide shift to a strict plant-based diet to prevent and reverse chronic disease.

The Animals Are Very Important

Being a vegan also eliminates *needless* cruelty to animals. I never heard of anyone say that slaughterhouses and meat-packing plants are kind and "humane" to animals (and to their workers), especially the limited number of people to whom I have spoken who have worked in them. There is not one scientific reason that we as humans *have to* eat a single bit of animal food to procreate, thrive, evolve, prevent disease, and be well as a human species. The only reasons we kill animals for food that I can think of are fivefold:

1. We are just used to doing it. It's part of our culture.
2. It's easier for some people to just eat more meat and go off grains all together. This eliminates a lot of their junk food containing excess sweet-fat calories. Some grain intolerant people will also feel much better and for many it's easier to

eliminate all grains than find the grain(s) that is causing the problem, as well as eat only whole grain products.

3. Well-meaning but uninformed people think we need to eat animal foods to survive and thrive as human beings.

4. People like the taste of meats.

5. There is a *large economy* centered on meat production.

I will repeat this one more time: There is no biological (evolutionary) reason any more that we *have to* eat meat to survive and thrive as a species in the modern world. There just isn't. So all this massive cruelty and suffering done to animals predominantly from factory farming is for no evolutionary purpose. It's for one or more of the five reasons just stated.

So before any of you meat eaters **misrepresent** *what I just said,* let's be very clear about what I've said: You can obviously be healthy eating small amounts of animal products, and most of the healthiest cultures in the world do it. What I did say, though, is that there is not a shred of scientific evidence that we *have to* eat another mouthful of animal foods to thrive and be well as a human species. Therefore, there is no need for this cruel process of mass meat production. None! And there is a lot of evidence that a well thought out, high micronutrient vegetable-rich, whole-food, unrefined vegan diet is exactly what the world needs right now as far as preventing and reversing the chronic disease taxing every country's healthcare system. Eliminating factory farming of animals for food consumption would also be a great thing for our environment in reducing greenhouse gases, conserving precious water resources, protecting our soil and rain forests, and reducing the spread of infectious diseases that come from the waste derived from the factory farming of billions of animals per year.

I will go one step further: Leave the fish in the ocean alone as well. We don't need to eat fish either. We can get our anti-inflammatory omega-3 fatty acids from the same places animals do: lots of green vegetation, sea vegetables, and some nuts and seeds. And, if needed, in supplements from plant sources of omega-3 fatty acids (alpha-linolenic acid—ALA, docosahexaenoic acid—DHA and eicosapentaenoic acid—EPA) which are now available.

As we continue to deplete fish stocks, as Dr. Jenkins stated in the Foreword to this book, not only will we lose species of fish but we will also affect the ecology of the ocean, which can only cause us harm. Secondly, if we try to remedy the situation with intensive fish farming to grow fish faster in cramped quarters, I predict unhealthy things will happen, as presently occurs with factory farming of animals for food.

Chapter 9

DOUBLE TROUBLE? DAIRY AND GRAINS

There are a lot of competing ideas out there about what is good for you and what isn't. This is particularly true when it comes to dairy products and grains, especially wheat. These two foods or food groups can cause lots of ill health. I could sum up my recommendations for the above in two simple statements:

- Don't eat dairy products in any shape or form from any animal. Do this 100 percent for *at least one month* (no cheese, ice cream, sour cream, milk, butter, cottage cheese, yogurt, kefir) or preferably for a lifetime. See how you feel.

- Eat only *whole* or *sprouted* grain products that you know you are NOT sensitive to. Be very cautious with wheat and other glutinous grains, or go gluten free for one month.

Why No Dairy?

It is very simple. I have seen more suffering from common health complaints stopped immediately by eliminating dairy products than any other single medical therapy. It is so obvious. All you have to do is go off dairy products completely for at least three weeks, then reintroduce them. Just see for yourself.

I have a list of scientific reasons why I think you should not eat dairy products. But don't even read them if you are so locked into the false belief that dairy products are good for you and you have to eat them for strong bones and protein. If I have made any sense so far in this book, and you think I am sincere and reasonably intelligent, then just take the "Ain't Got Milk" challenge for one month and see for yourself. It will be abundantly clear that many of you will feel better, and many complaints—some mild, some serious—will be eliminated. When I say the "Ain't Got Milk" challenge, I mean all dairy products (milk, cheese, yogurt, ice cream, kefir, etc.) from any animal for one month.

Common Problems Improved with Dairy Elimination

This a *short list* of symptoms and conditions I have seen caused or aggravated by dairy products over the last three decades:

- Asthma
- Back pain
- Bedwetting
- Bloating
- Chronic cough, morning cough
- Chronic infections of the sinuses, ears, or throat
- Constipation (sometimes diarrhea)
- Edema – water retention
- Foggy brain
- Headaches (migraines)
- Hearing problems in young children (fluid in ears)
- Heartburn (GERD)
- Joint pain (any joint)
- Menstrual cramps
- Nasal congestion
- Puffy hands and fingers
- Rashes
- Sleep apnea
- Snoring
- Stomach pain, cramping

- Upper respiratory phlegm production
- Water retention
- Weight excess

Sometimes when I tell people to avoid all dairy products for a month or two, they look at me with this incredulous look, as if I had just said the most un-American thing I could ever say. But I'm not kidding. The first three weeks will be hard, but then the cravings will go away. I am not sure why the cravings last three weeks, but that has been my observation with milk products, especially cheeses. The harder and more ridiculous this concept of staying off milk products seems to you, the more I want you to try it! The most "stunned" people are usually the ones who have the most dramatic responses. Make sure you note any symptoms or bodily changes that occur while off dairy products and then pay attention to what happens when you add them back into your diet. (Use the Diet-Exercise-Symptom Diary under Educational Handouts at Prescription2000.com to chart symptoms.)

Where's Calcium for my Bones?

I know one thing you're thinking: "How do I get calcium for my bones if I am off dairy products?" In America, we are hammered with the "calcium-milk-bone myth" from an early age.

A paper in 2009 in the well-respected *American Journal of Clinical Nutrition* by Dr. Amy Joy Lanou challenges this very issue of dairy products and bone loss-fracture prevention. Commenting on two very large studies, she states, "Both showed no protective effect of increased milk consumption on fracture risk." And she continues, "Further, two meta-analyses of studies of milk or dairy consumption and fracture risk have shown no reduction in risk with higher intakes of milk, dairy, or total dietary calcium."[1]

It is noted that osteoporotic bone fracture rates are highest in countries that consume the most dairy, calcium, and animal protein.[2] This article is a must-read. It notes that the countries with the highest calcium intakes have the highest hip fracture rates and those with the lowest calcium intake have the lowest. Fracture risk is associated with higher protein intake, which can cause more calcium spill in the urine.[3] Dr. Lanou has co-authored (with Michael Castleman) an easily read and incredibly well-referenced book on this very topic, which I highly recommend (*Building Bone Vitality*, 2009) if you are fearful of your bones falling apart by not eating dairy products.

To be balanced on the protein and urine loss of calcium debate, a counter to this argument was expressed in an interview I did with Dr. Loren Cordain, author of the *Paleo Diet* (2011). He states that while higher animal protein intakes can increase calcium loss in the urine, higher meat diets also increase calcium absorption, thereby resulting in a net increase in calcium absorption. He further states that increased meat consumption enhances IGF-1 which can increase bone formation by stimulating the bone forming cells called osteocytes.[4]

Of course, there are successfully aging cultures that eat natural dairy products and do fine. Take for instance the "Blue Zone" Sardinian (Italy) goat and sheep herders. Because these are naturally free-ranged animals, they probably have a more anti-inflammatory fatty acid profile (more omega-3 fatty acids), and goats in particular consume a plant (dwarf curry) rich in a powerful anti-inflammatory compound called arzanol. The popular goat milk and cheese products consumed by Sardinians may have healthful anti-inflammatory properties from the good fatty acid profile and arzanol.[5]

Generally speaking, healthy aging cultures from around the world consume small quantities of dairy products. Eating dairy naturally and locally is considerably different from eating mass-produced, pasteurized dairy products from factory farming in which the animals are given hormones and antibiotics, live in crowded conditions, and are kept in nearly a year-round state of lactation. Also, the diets of these healthy aging cultures are generally not high animal protein diets. They are generally low to moderate in animal protein with lots of vegetables, beans, and a staple starch, fruit, some nuts and seeds, virtually no processed foods, and lots of physical activity and sunshine (vitamin D).[6] Their diets are generally more alkaline from lots of vegetables and fruit and less animal foods and virtually no processed foods. Therefore they are more calcium sparing. Grains, even whole grains, are mildly acidic, like meats, which may aggravate bone loss if not balanced by a high intake of fruits and vegetables.

Consider the following facts and then decide for yourself whether dairy products really do your body good, or just eliminate them completely for one month and see how you feel:

- Humans are the only species to regularly consume the milk of another species after weaning.
- Increasing milk (dairy products) consumption has not consistently been shown to improve bone density and reduce fracture risk.[7]
- Cheeses, especially hard cheeses, are some of the most acid-producing foods, which contribute to bone loss by taking calcium and phosphorous from bone to buffer the blood.[8]
- Prostate cancer and possibly ovarian cancer have been linked to dairy products.[9]
- Many people are lactose intolerant, meaning that they cannot digest the sugar in milk. (This is not a true allergy but rather an enzyme deficiency.) This can cause lots of G.I. complaints.[10]
- Dairy products can be high in saturated fat and cholesterol generally.[11]
- Dairy products are not an adequate source of vitamin D, with current research suggesting 1,000–5,000 IU per day being more optimal.[12]
- Feeding infants cow's milk early in life may increase the risk of type 1 diabetes by triggering an autoimmune reaction.[13]
- Milk proteins, milk sugar, fat, and unsaturated fat in dairy products can increase health risks for children, such as obesity, diabetes, and heart disease.[14]
- The American Academy of Pediatrics recommends that infants below one year of age not be given whole cow's milk.[15]
- Early introduction of milk in children may increase the risk of constipation and iron deficiency.[16]

- There are many food-intolerant reactions to dairy products. You name a symptom, and I have seen it caused by some type of dairy product consumption.

- The Paleolithic diet, which many people seem excited about, didn't contain any dairy products at all (except maybe occasional eggs), yet where is the evidence that Paleolithic man had weak bones and wasn't strong?

- Species with the most massive bone structure (elephants, hippos, rhinos, giraffes, cows, etc.) don't eat milk products to maintain strong bones or muscle mass.

You don't have to take my word for it any more than you have to believe the slogans of the dairy councils or those world-famous athletes with the milk mustaches, which in my opinion did a great disservice to the public. Why not just go with how your body feels? Take one month and do the "Ain't Got Milk" challenge and completely eliminate *all dairy products*. Don't just cut down or cut out one group of dairy products. Go off *all* dairy products from all species of animals for one month. Keep a Diet-Symptom-Exercise Diary (see Educational Handouts at Prescription2000.com) and notice how many symptoms improve. After one month, add back in the dairy products you ate most frequently and see how you feel. Many people will recognize that dairy causes some distressing symptoms. Some will also notice that dairy is a cause of excess calories, resulting in weight gain.

Problems with Dairy Product Elimination

Some simple and fixable problems can occur when "big" dairy consumers go off dairy products. Some experience a drop in blood sugar because they have such a limited diet and don't know what else to eat. This is solved by eating whole, unprocessed foods frequently off the Basic Elimination Diet (BED) food list. Others may get leg cramps, especially at night, because they do not eat other sources of calcium and magnesium. They might take a calcium/ magnesium supplement or better yet eat calcium and magnesium-rich plant foods (greens). If you continue to eat a higher meat protein diet, you may have to take more calcium when stopping dairy products to balance the calcium spill triggered by the higher meat intake.

Grains—Why the Controversy?

Since standing agriculture is only about ten thousand years old, grain consumption is relatively new on the human evolutionary scene.[17] As we discussed in the last chapter, our simian ancestors were tree dwellers, eating vegetation and fruit. Our Paleolithic ancestors may have only had some wild grains to chew on. So grains weren't a significant part of their diet, if at all. Some people think that for those "evolutionary reasons," grains are something we shouldn't eat; others think whole grain is a perfect fuel source.

What we can say about this controversy is that most successful aging populations around the world consume some type of staple grain product on a regular basis. The Okinawan Centenarians (Okinawa, Japan) consume white and brown rice, wheat (udon), millet, and buckwheat (soba) noodles; Sardinians (Italy) consume wheat bread; Nicoyans (Costa Rica) consume calcium- and magnesium-rich corn (maize) tortillas and rice; Hunzans (Pakistan) consume a variety of whole grains (wheat, millet, barley, buckwheat); Vilcabambans (Ecuador) consume whole grains, corn, quinoa, wheat, and barley; Abkhasians (part of northern Georgia; formerly part of the USSR) consume a cornmeal mash called *abista*; and Seventh Day Adventists (United States) consume whole grains.[18]

The grains eaten by these people provide optimal fuel to support their daily hard work and activity. Grains are also cheap and easy to produce. If these healthy cultures can eat these grains, then they can't be bad for you in the way and form in which these populations consume them.

Why Eat Grains?

Grains, especially in their whole state, are an excellent source of time-released carbohydrates, along with fiber, vitamins, minerals, essential fatty acids, and, yes, even protein. They are a perfect food on paper in their *whole, unrefined state* as long as: (1) you don't have an intolerance to that grain, which a significant number of people do, and (2) if the grains you consume are whole grains and don't have sweet-fat calories added to them, including hydrogenated vegetable oils, trans-fats, and added calorie sweeteners.

What's so Good about Whole Grains?

Whole grains are good sources of fiber, vitamins, minerals, good fatty acids, beneficial phytochemicals, and time-released sugars. Unlike "white" refined grains, they contain the outer fiber layer and the nutrient-rich germ, as well as the starchy endosperm, which is all that is left in the refined grain.

Diets that contain at least three or more ounce equivalents of whole grains per day may help with weight control and can reduce the risk of several chronic diseases, such as coronary heart disease and some kinds of cancer.[19]

In addition, whole grain products tend not to be found in confectionary foods that have added fats, oils, and sugars, or what I call "sweet-fat calories." Since they have the fiber and germ, unlike a refined grain product, they tend to be more filling and usually have a slower blood sugar release, both of which are good for weight control and chronic disease prevention.

Do this experiment. Get a loaf of real *whole-* or *sprouted-grain* bread. Remember, one of those two words is the first word(s) after *Ingredients* on the package label. True whole or sprouted grain bread is generally not fortified. Get a white flour baguette. See which bread you can eat more of. Maybe at best you can eat two or maybe three slices of the sprouted or whole-grain bread. Most of you will only eat one piece. At another time, go for the baguette.

Some of you, like me, might be able to eat the whole baguette in a sitting or by the time I get done grocery shopping! Even if the calories and glycemic response were the same, you will eat more of the refined grain product because they are less filling and can cause more "carb" cravings.

What Exactly Is a Whole Grain?

There is no universally accepted definition of whole-grain foods, and labels may be hard to understand. Labels like "wheat bread," "stone-ground," and "seven-grain bread" do not guarantee that the food contains whole grains. Color is not a good indicator of whole grains either, because foods may be darker simply because of added molasses or food coloring.[20] I tell patients to look at the first words right after the word "Ingredients" on the label. If the first words are "whole grain" or "sprouted grain," it is a predominantly whole-grain product and you are good to go. If the bread is enriched with vitamins or minerals, it is generally not a whole-grain product or has only a small amount of whole grain and generally should be avoided.

The U.S. Dietary Guidelines use the American Association of Cereal Chemists' definition, which is: "Foods made from the entire grain seed, usually called the kernel, which consists of the *bran*, *germ*, and *endosperm*. If the kernel has been cracked, crushed, or flaked, it must retain nearly the same relative proportions of bran, germ, and endosperm as the original grain in order to be called whole grain."[21]

The U.S. Food and Drug Administration (FDA), on the other hand, only requires foods that bear the whole grain health claim to: *(1) contain 51 percent or more whole-grain ingredients by weight per reference amount and (2) be low in fat.*[22]

Anatomy of a Whole Grain Kernel

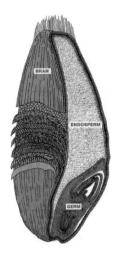

Bran: Protective outer layer rich in insoluble fiber, B vitamins, trace minerals, and phytonutrients. About 14% of the kernel by weight. Removed with refining.

Endosperm: Sometimes called the kernel, is primarily an energy source providing carbohydrates and protein. It contains smaller amounts of B vitamins, iron and soluble fiber. About 83% of the kernel by weight. This portion of the kernel remains in refined grain products.

Germ: Is the nutrient-rich embryo of the seed. It is a concentrated source of nutrients including B vitamins, vitamin E, fatty acids, antioxidants and phytonutrients. Less than 3% of the kernel by weight. It is removed in refined grains.

Source of kernel image: Montana Wheat and Barley Committee. Montana's Official State website. http://wbc.agr.mt.gov/Consumers/diagram_kernel.html (accessed Feb. 26, 2011).

Americans have been consuming more grain products in the last thirty to forty years, but only fifteen percent are whole grains while eighty-five percent are refined grains. This is a prescription for excess calories, weight gain, and chronic disease since many of these refined grain products come with extra sweet-fat calories. This consumption of refined grains also gives all carbohydrates a bad name, which is a disservice to the public's health. [23]

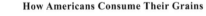

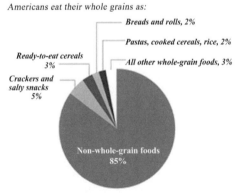

How Americans Consume Their Grains

Americans eat their whole grains as:

- Breads and rolls, 2%
- Pastas, cooked cereals, rice, 2%
- All other whole-grain foods, 3%
- Ready-to-eat cereals 3%
- Crackers and salty snacks 5%
- Non-whole-grain foods 85%

Source: ERS analysis of 1999-2000 National Health and Nutrition Examination Survey (NHANES) Data.

Why Aren't We Eating Whole Grains?

There are a few reasons: They cost more; they take longer to cook; they are not available in most restaurants when we eat out; they initially don't taste as good to many people; and they are not easily available in regular grocery stores.

One of the great things about living in a modern urban setting in the United States is that stores like Trader Joe's, Whole Foods Market, natural food co-ops, and health food sections in regular grocery stores now make it easy to get whole-grain products. This is a good thing about the modern lifestyle: If we consumers buy it, it will be on the shelves. If we don't buy the refined flour products, eventually they will go away. It's up to us. Here is capitalism at its best: Be educated. Buy mostly whole- or sprouted-grain products, and those are the nutritious and wholesome foods that will be stocked in grocery stores. Consequently, our health will improve.

Grain Intolerance

Sooner or later, I have to appear to contradict myself and confuse you. Otherwise, I wouldn't be a good author and health "expert." Here goes. Even if everyone in the United States switched over to eating whole or sprouted grains 100 percent overnight, there would be a significant group of people who wouldn't feel well. They would have some type of intolerance to the grain, especially with wheat, possibly the other glutinous grains (oat, barley, rye), and corn as well.

Some individuals would just not feel well until they go off most grains. That is why I came up with the Basic Elimination Diet (BED) (Appendix A). Though I am adamant about everyone taking a one-month trial off *all* dairy products, a grain-free diet except for brown rice and other non-glutinous grains would be an excellent idea and result in noted symptom improvement in many individuals.

While I have experienced many patients with grain intolerance in almost three decades of clinical practice, usually from refined wheat products in confectionary foods and breads, and

I have read and heard through interviews the arguments on the adverse health consequences of cereal grains from such respected researchers as Dr. Loren Cordain (*The Paleo Diet*, 2011), [24] I still feel strongly that whole grains have to and can be part of a healthy human diet for most of humanity. We need cereal grains as an energy and protein source for the expanding world population. If we eat grains in their whole state only, we will eliminate the refined grains and confectionary foods that bring along with them extra added calories from fats, oils, and sugars, as well as a poor glycemic response that increase our risk to chronic diseases. If we are aware of the potential for grain intolerance (especially from glutinous grains) as educated health consumers and as intelligent health practitioners, the adverse effects of grain intolerance can be kept to a minimum. Lastly, if we consume whole grains as part of a whole unprocessed, predominantly plant foods diet with a wide variety of protective phytochemicals from vegetables, fruit, beans, nuts and seeds, we will do fine. As I have mentioned previously, if the most functional and healthy aging Blue Zone cultures with low incidences of chronic diseases have grains as part of their diets, then we can to. In addition the modern era allows us immediate and easy access to so many more nutrient-dense foods of plant origin than in the Neolithic era, where man may have been limited to certain staple grains and a small variety of root crops for his daily subsistence. We should take advantage of this and create dietary choices that bring us the greatest amount of micronutrients per calorie of food intake and subsequent optimal health.

Chapter 10

THE BIG THREE: ALCOHOL, CAFFEINE, AND SUGAR

What do alcohol, caffeine, and sugar have in common?
They are all:

- consumed by large portions of the population;
- very addictive;
- easily abused;
- mood altering and can cause depression;
- fatigue inducing;
- low in nutrient density;
- contributors to ill health if consumed in large amounts, especially in conjunction with processed food diets and modern-day stressful living;
- substances which must be used in moderation in order for excellent health to be maintained.

Almost no food substance in moderation is harmful. Likewise, almost any food in excess, except for maybe vegetables, is harmful. The big three—alcohol, caffeine, and sugar—are very difficult for many to use in moderation, and any one in excess can be very destructive to health. Periodic abstinence from these foods, even for one or two days a week, can keep you in control and prevent these foods from getting the upper hand on your health. This is especially true in fast-paced modern life where these addictive food components can lead our diet and our bodies into health patterns where we really should not go.

Alcohol

Alcohol consumption is associated with a reduced risk in heart disease at approximately one drink in females and two drinks in males, per day.[1] In Western culture, you have to be careful that you don't use this as an excuse to consume excess calories! A gram of alcohol is usually seven calories (fat = 9 cal; protein = 4 cal; carb = 4 cal). Then there are the added calories from how the alcohol is made and what you mix it with. Alcohol is a relatively "empty" calorie source.

Yes, there is resveratrol, a potent antioxidant and popular "anti-aging" compound found in red wine, and compounds in hops from beer that may improve insulin resistance or reduce menopausal symptoms, but I wouldn't call alcohol a nutrient-dense food.

The way we use alcohol in our busy, modern lives needs a bit of caution. We usually use it to unwind or de-stress at the end of a hectic day. I would have no problem with this if you were lean and had finished thirty to sixty minutes of aerobic exercise and some strength and flexibility exercise as well. This would not be a problem either if you were having a "light" soup and salad or a small meal of lean animal protein, a good starch, and lots of vegetables in the evening at about five o'clock. That is not most people's reality.

Americans often eat late (seven to nine o'clock at night after a very stressful day), have a few drinks, eat a big, calorie-rich meal, and veg out in front of the television. Yes, this is a generalization, but you get the idea. We are throwing alcohol on top of a stressful day, where most people weren't physically active, and we are mixing it with a late dinner of excess calories.

What I see in practice is that when patients who have been regular daily consumers cut out alcohol, there is usually an easy five- to ten-pound weight loss that first month without trying. Maybe some of that is the food that goes along with the alcohol consumption? I don't know.

Drinking in the evening, though it may relax you, really can cause problems with lethargy, fatigue, or "fogginess" that evening and the next morning as well. If I had a dollar for every time someone said the fog cleared in the morning after eliminating a nighttime food or alcoholic drink, I'd be rich.

My goal for you in practicing periodic abstinence from alcohol is that you really know how it affects your life and that you are in control of it—not the other way around. In fact, that is my goal for you regarding all food intake.

Caffeine: The Legal Drug

Caffeine is a very addictive substance. It is a legal drug, in my opinion (I use it). What makes it dangerous in this busy, modern society is that it is a vehicle for unwanted calories (sugar and fat), takes the place of good calories, and in the context of a poor diet and busy lifestyle can cause blood sugar fluctuations resulting in energy, cognition, and mood problems that can really run a person's life—in the wrong direction.

The world of caffeine drinks is intertwined with every age group and all aspects of modern life. The current "energy drink revolution" is a prime example. Young teenagers can get hooked on caffeine without ever drinking a cup of coffee at home in front of their parents. I also cringe when I see parents buying heavily sweetened, sugar-laden, dairy-containing, espresso-loaded coffee drinks with a refined flour, sweet-fat muffin or something of that nature for their child or teenager. Not good! You are not doing the child any favors. Coffee shops, and I frequent them regularly, are places where bad health habits can be created and perpetuated. They are legal drug houses; Sugar, fat, refined grains, dairy, and caffeine are the drugs.

Caffeine Doesn't like Being Alone!

Caffeine drinks usually come with other things. Caffeine in coffee drinks come with a lot of calories because of the dairy products, chocolate, syrups, or other added sweeteners (sucrose from cane or beet sugar). A day or two per week or every month or so individuals should be caffeine free for a few days so you can remember how you feel being off caffeine. The goal is for you to be in control of the drug. If you don't know how you feel off it, it's hard to make conscious choices.

I often share this visualization with my patients. It is one thing to have a large breakfast and coffee and then go out and do manual labor for a day, let's say in an agrarian society. It is totally another to be racing out of the house, stressed, going through the drive-thru to get a whipped cream-topped, chocolate, and sugar-filled coffee drink, maybe eating a muffin on the way to dropping off the kids at school and then going to work. The former example will do no harm. The latter example is a prescription for exhaustion, head-aches, anxiety, mood changes, and a variety of other symptoms.

What people don't understand is that regular coffee (or caf-feine) consumption leads to a withdrawal phase every twenty-four hours.[2] By withdrawal phase, I don't mean the sometimes vicious headaches you can get when you stop caffeine cold turkey. I mean you are just sitting there in your office or at home and you feel a bit down, and you just want that coffee or caffeine drink at the same time the next day; it almost seems as if for no reason.

A counter-intuitive reality is that if you chronically ingest a lot of caffeine, especially with sugar, you can create depression and fatigue.[3] This becomes evident after four to seven days of being caffeine and sugar free and your energy and mood begin to return.

Caffeine and Calorie Content of Coffee Drinks

When you are in your local coffee establishment, ask or look for their nutrition fact sheet or brochure. You will be amazed how many calories (four to five hundred) are in one of the fancy coffee drinks; and in a tall or large cup of plain coffee, the caffeine content can be three to four hundred milligrams! The goal is to be aware and in control of your intake.

Caffeine-Related Problems

Here are a number of health conditions that may improve with coffee or caffeine elimination or reduction:[4]

- Abdominal pain or discomfort of unknown cause
- Anxiety, irritability, and nervousness
- Arthritis
- Autoimmune disorders
- Colitis, diverticulitis, diarrhea, and other irritable bowel symptoms
- Chronic Fatigue Syndrome
- Depression
- Dizziness, Meniere's syndrome, or tinnitus (ringing in the ears)
- Fibrocystic breast disease
- Gout (elevated uric acid levels)
- Heart disease or heart palpitations
- High blood pressure
- High cholesterol
- Hypoglycemia (low blood sugar)
- Indigestion/heartburn
- Insomnia and interrupted or poor-quality sleep
- Liver disease and gallbladder problems such as gallstones
- Kidney or bladder problems, including kidney stones
- Migraines or other vascular headaches
- Muscle pain
- Osteoporosis
- Skin irritations, rashes, and dryness
- Ulcers, heartburn, and stomach problems such as hiatal hernias
- Urinary tract irritation

Caffeine Conclusions: Controlling This Legal Drug

The reason I have spent so much time on caffeine use and abuse is because I see its adverse affect on people's lives on a daily basis. I have seen it affect mine. For short periods, I have let it get the best of me. If not controlled, caffeine excess from coffee, tea, sodas, energy drinks, and some medications can lead you to some significant health problems treated symptomatically with medication and unnecessary medical tests. All this suffering, money, and time might be totally avoided with awareness and control of this legal drug. Take a caffeine break weekly. Just that can help you be in control of your health a bit more, which is what this book is all about.

Sugar—Friend or Foe?

Sugars are the simplest form of carbohydrates. Carbohydrates are important to all living things with regard to storage and transport of energy and structure. The common term "sugar" refers mainly to sucrose or table sugar. Sugar primarily comes from sugar cane and sugar beets, but it also comes from fruit, honey, sorghum, maple syrup, and other sources.

Sugar in itself can't be bad. Every cell needs it. We evolved searching daily for calories and sweet things. More often than not, there wasn't enough. Our bodies have evolved to being very efficient at storing energy to be used later (referred to as the "Thrifty Gene Hypothesis").[5] The natural sugars we came in contact with were from fruit mainly, and possibly some honey. Other sugars we consumed were stored as complex sugars or starches in plants such as root vegetables or maybe wild grains. All of these sugars came with protective plant compounds, phytonutrients, antioxidants, vitamins, minerals, and fiber, and because they were in the context of the whole food, they were released slower or had what is called a "lower glycemic response," which is associated with greater health.

Today we sit on our behinds at home or in our cars. Food can either be driven to us or we can drive up to the food. The added sugars in foods, whether from cane or beet (sucrose) or high fructose corn syrup, are totally unnecessary for our survival. What's more, these added sweeteners contain neither phytochemicals, fiber nor nutrients to help metabolize the extra calories and protect our bodies from internal and external insults, nor important plant compounds to give our genes the right message about proper cellular functioning. The excess calories have to go somewhere, especially since we aren't burning them off, so they get stored as fat. In turn, fat and excess calories lead to inflammation and we get more chronic disease. Excess sugar can also increase cholesterol.

Humans most commonly add sucrose, a disaccharide (glucose and fructose), as their main sweetener. Commercially produced table sugar (sucrose) comes either from sugar cane or from sugar beet. Corn sweeteners, such as high fructose corn syrup (HFCS), are the most common added sweeteners in processed foods. The term HFCS actually refers to any of a group of corn syrups (pure glucose, a monosaccharide) that have undergone enzymatic processing to increase the fructose (monosaccharide) content. The enzymatically enhanced corn syrup, now fructose, is mixed with pure corn syrup, which is 100 percent glucose, in varying percentages, and is found virtually in all processed foods and beverages, including soft drinks, cookies, crackers, salad dressings, snack foods, soups, etc. *Even if these sugars were metabolized perfectly by our bodies with no adverse effects, they are totally unnecessary and are only added calories.* The most common types of high fructose corn syrup are:[6]

- HFCS 90—approximately 90 percent fructose and 10 percent glucose, made in small quantities mainly to increase the fructose content of HFCS 42 to 55.
- HFCS 55—approximately 55 percent fructose and 45 percent glucose, primarily used in soft drinks.
- HFCS 42—approximately 42 percent fructose and 58 percent glucose, mainly used in foods and baked goods.

High fructose corn syrup has given fruit a bad rap because "fructose" is fruit sugar, so many people are paranoid about eating fruit. As you can see, though, HFCS has varying amounts of fructose and glucose to create the desired sweetness for a product. The fructose in a piece of fruit is held in the complex of water, fiber, and phytochemicals, so with fruit your body is getting less of a sugar load as well as a slower release of the sugar and more protective compounds with it. My point? *Don't be paranoid of whole fruit.* Have at it! It's so good for you. Try not to consume processed foods in general with any kind of added sugars. Period. The debate of whether added HFCS is better or worse for you than added table sugar (sucrose) is a moot point. *We shouldn't be eating a lot of foods that have either one of these totally unnecessary added calorie sweeteners in the first place.*

Sugar in Natural Food: Is it Better?

Natural sugars come in fruit, grains, legumes, and vegetables. Since natural sugars are a calorie source when consumed in excess, they can increase weight and inflammation like other calories. But it is harder to eat excess calories when eating whole, unprocessed foods with no added sugars of any type.

In general, natural sugars are better than "added" manufactured sugars because they come in a complex of fiber and other phytonutrients that slow the release of these sugars into our bodies, making the metabolism of the sugar less stressful to our endocrine (adrenal glands, liver, pancreas, brain) organs over time. Nutrients that come with these natural sugars in complex whole foods assist in the metabolism of that sugar instead of taking those nutrients from body stores needed for this and other important bodily processes.

The truth is sucrose, or table sugar (fructose and glucose), and high fructose corn syrup (fructose and glucose) are metabolized similarly and, in small amounts don't cause disease any more than natural sugars found in whole foods. But—and this is a big but—*there is no need for these two types of sugars to be added to our food supply (adding to our total caloric load) AT ALL for human survival and optimal functioning. And these two unnecessary calorie sweeteners are added to most refined foods and drinks which we consume large quantities of in this country. This does affect our collective health significantly and adversely.*

Bottom line: If you just eat whole, unprocessed foods (real foods!), you cut out the unnecessary calories from these added calorie sweeteners or sugars. You also cut out the stress to the organs that have to process these added sugars (adrenals, liver, and pancreas). These extra sugar calories are just not necessary— period! Excess sugar equals excess calories and inflammation, which are both very harmful to our health. It is so simple. Just eat whole foods (vegetables, fruit, beans, raw nuts and seeds, and whole grains) and you don't have to read a label or worry about added sugars.

Sugar's Job: Get into the Cell and be "Burned"

Sugar's role is to be burned as energy in the cell. If that happens efficiently, without a glitch, life works well. If insulin, the doorman of the cell, can't unlock or open the door for any reason, known or unknown, sugar can't get into the cell, and bad things start to happen.

On the outside of the cell, if sugar in the bloodstream starts to elevate, an excess of blood sugar can cause a variety of long-term ill effects to the body, slowly damaging blood vessels, nerves, eyes, and kidneys, and actually *increase the aging process*. With the rise in blood sugar, insulin keeps being secreted by the pancreas to try to open the door of the cell to get sugar into the cell to be burned as energy.

If the sugar is a simple sugar, it generally gets absorbed rapidly, causing the pancreas to respond quickly, which it does very well. There is quick demand for insulin. If, over time, this process challenges those cells in the pancreas enough, they start to wear out and fail to produce insulin adequately. The person might eventually develop insulin-dependent diabetes (meaning they have to take insulin shots to lower their blood sugar). But first, this person might develop what is called "insulin resistance."

Sugar and Insulin Resistance

The chronic ingestion of any added sugars that lead to excess calories can aggravate insulin resistance. Excess calories, weight, and excess fat in the cell (intramyocellular fat) can all increase the risk of insulin resistance, leading to higher circulating insulin (and blood sugar) levels. So while it is important to eat low glycemic carbohydrates, it's also important to keep your total calorie and fat levels down to improve insulin resistance.

Excess insulin can also increase cholesterol.[7] So eating sugar could indirectly increase cholesterol and cardiovascular risk. High insulin levels also increase fat storage.

Insulin is an inflammatory hormone. Since almost all chronic diseases (heart disease, cancer, diabetes, bone loss, stroke, hypertension, and degenerative eye and brain disorders) come from excessive inflammation, excessive insulin is not a good thing. Insulin is also a growth-promoting hormone, so aside from increasing inflammation it can also increase the risk of cancer.

Bottom line: if you control your blood sugar (fasting < 90 mg/dl, some say < 80 mg/dl is optimal) and keep you insulin low (<10 uU/ml, some say lower), you reduce your risk of chronic inflammatory diseases and slow the aging process.

Staying Healthy "Pearl" about Sugar

One common point that is a true belief of every dietary philosophy I know, from raw food veganism to the high-fat, high-protein diet proponents, and everything in between: The goal of all diets is to control blood sugar (and insulin) levels for optimal health and chronic disease prevention and/or reversal. Every diet guru agrees on this. And it is correct. Controlling blood sugar and insulin levels—sometimes called "good glycemic control"—increases optimal function and slows the aging process. That is why almost any diet philosophy can work if you use the diet to achieve this goal. Ideally, you want to control blood sugar and insulin levels at a calorie level that allows you to stay lean but provides you with the maximum amount of vitamins, minerals, and phytonutrients to protect you and optimize your metabolism. I hate to be repetitive, folks, but that's a micronutrient-rich, plant-strong, unprocessed vegan diet.

Sugar and Your Intestines

Undigested simple sugars can go into the bowel, and bacteria—generally in the large intestine—can work on these sugars and produce gas and bloating or more complex chemicals called organic acids that can have extra intestinal effects (other places in the body). Similar symptoms may occur with undigested simple sugars increasing fungal growth.

Cutting out all refined sugars and sometimes even whole unprocessed sugars from foods and drink can dramatically reduce gut symptoms and sometimes systemic problems (headaches, joint pain, etc.). Adding a good probiotic (good bacteria) along with antifungal treatment may also provide additional benefit. Some people need stool exams to see if there is any bacterial (or fungal) overgrowth to be treated. Sometimes I give a short course of antibiotics for antibiotic sensitive bacteria I find in a stool exam, which is overgrown in the gut.

Some individuals with carbohydrate sensitivity need to go on the Specific Carbohydrate Diet (SCD), which is explained in detail by the late Elaine Gottschall in her book *Breaking the Vicious Cycle: Intestinal Health Through Diet*. The SCD allows for carbohydrates that require minimal digestion and are completely absorbed (honey and fruit are acceptable, but no grains, beans, starchy vegetables, or dairy products except hard cheeses). This leaves no sugars for the intestinal bacteria to feed on and produce unwanted gas and metabolites. This diet has also been used with success in some autistic children as part of an overall treatment strategy.[8]

Sugars and Your Hormones

The simplest way to give your hormones a break when it comes to sugar consumption is to eat it either as whole fruit or intact in legumes, vegetables, nuts and seeds, and/or whole grains. These forms of complex sugars put less stress on your adrenal glands, pancreas, and liver, producing a smoother blood sugar rise and fall.

The popular term is to eat *low glycemic* foods. Usually, but not always, low glycemic foods are found in whole, unrefined plant foods, especially beans, lentils, peas, and some pastas. Yes, I said pastas! Most pastas have a better glycemic index than breads. Of course eat whole grain pastas when you can. Shoot for eating low glycemic, unprocessed carbohydrate-rich foods (GI < 55; glycemicindex.com).

Sugar and Your Brain

Your brain doesn't like to be without two things for too long: oxygen and sugar. A lack of either can cause mental fogginess, difficulty thinking, irritability, or even headaches in some.

Your brain cells use more than twice the energy as other cells in your body. Neurons require high energy because they're always working metabolically. Even during sleep, neurons are repairing and rebuilding. Neurons manufacture enzymes and neurotransmitters that are transported to the ends of their nerve branches, which takes energy. Nerve transmission is a very energy-intensive use of glucose, consuming one-half of all the brain's energy (nearly 10 percent of the whole body's energy).[9]

Thinking can be exhausting. Glucose can be rapidly used up during mental activity. Reduced amounts of glucose can impair acetylcholine synthesis, which is an important neurotransmitter in the brain for memory.[10]

A sugary snack or soft drink that quickly raises your blood sugar level can give you a boost, especially if it has caffeine added to it, but this is generally for a short period of time. As previously mentioned, when you eat something that causes a rapid rise in your blood sugar, your pancreas secretes a burst of insulin. Subsequently the glucose available to your brain drops sometime later. Neurons, which can't store glucose, experience energy deprivation (hypoglycemia). Hours later, you can feel foggy-brained, weak, confused, and/or nervous. Your ability to focus and think is impaired. Low blood glucose levels can lead to a significant deterioration in attention abilities. The goal again is to eat slow-release sugars (low glycemic foods) to give your brain a constant flow of energy.[11]

Sugar Cravings: Simple Things You Can Do

Here are a few suggestions for dealing with those nasty sugar cravings:

- First and foremost, eat whole food. Don't eat refined and processed foods.
- Eat three meals with whole-food snacks in between if you are hungry. The carbohydrates you eat should be in their whole, unrefined state: whole fruit, beans (and bean spreads), lentil, peas, pastas, whole/sprouted grains, root vegetables such as yams, sweet potatoes, and nuts and seeds.
- Don't use added sweeteners of any kind.
- Don't skip meals! Have a whole-food snack available when you get hungry.
- Only have whole foods in your refrigerator, in your cupboards, and at work. Under stress or if you just want to eat for any reason, just have whole foods available in your immediate surroundings and eat them.
- Avoid stimulants, especially when they are sugar-laden, such as soft drinks or complex coffee drinks. Only have caffeine in coffee or tea with a meal or some kind of whole food. You might give up caffeine for a while to make it easier.
- Get regular aerobic exercise daily. If you are going to eat a sweet, exercise right afterward.
- Do strength training to build lean muscle. Lean muscle helps keep blood sugar low.

Here are some basic blood sugar-stabilizing nutrients (*these are much less important than* **correcting your diet**, yet they still can help; these are also available over the counter):

- Glutamine: 3,000–5,000 mg/d between meals
- Free-form amino acid powder between meals
- 5-HTP: 100–300 mg at 4:00 p.m. and at bedtime on an empty stomach (tryptophan→5HTP→serotonin→melatonin)
- A good high-potency multivitamin/mineral
- A good B-complex (B50s–B100s)
- Extra B1: 100–300 mg/d until sugar cravings are gone
- B5: 1,000–3,000 mg/d especially if adrenal fatigue is suggested
- Vitamin C: 1,000–4,000 mg/d
- Vitamin D: 2,000–5,000 IU/d
- Chromium: 400–1,000 mcg/d with food
- Magnesium: 200–400 mg/d
- Zinc: 20–30 mg/d

How Not to Worry about Sugar

Eat whole food and lots of it! Several times per day when hungry. This is the real key. Eat! Make sure you are eating *whole, unprocessed*, carbohydrate-rich, protein adequate, nutrient-dense foods with lots of phytochemicals and fiber when you eat them. Avoid stimulants (e.g., caffeine, energy drinks, soft drinks), especially sweetened stimulants. And as always, exercise, build lean muscle, and move your body daily!

Chapter 11

FOOD INTOLERANCE AND ALLERGIES

Food intolerance and allergies are somewhat ignored by traditional nutrition circles. While I talk about improving the health of the United States and the world by changing macronutrition or by eating different food groups, these facts don't take into account the role of food intolerance on quality of individual life.

Making broad, sweeping dietary and lifestyle changes, as I have mentioned throughout the book, if implemented, will have great benefits to society. Some individuals, while reducing their risk of the major chronic diseases, may not feel well, or will have certain symptoms or conditions aggravated on a whole-food diet because of food sensitivities. The most glaring example is usually wheat consumption and food intolerance, assuming you already got rid of all milk products!

Some people believe that wheat, whole grain or not, is a greater problem than dairy products from a food intolerance point of view. It is high on my list as well. Ideally, I would love all my patients to go off all dairy, wheat (and glutinous grains), added sugars, caffeine drinks, and alcohol for a month or two and eat a diet of whole, mainly plant-based foods. You would see a great deal of improvement in a lot of people and relief from a lot of different complaints.

Over the years, I have seen wheat do almost as much "damage" as dairy products. Name the symptom, and I have seen it caused by wheat intolerance. Wheat sensitivity could also be caused by celiac disease, which is a severe form of intolerance to the gluten in the wheat that, if gone unnoticed, can result in severe malnutrition and bowel, joint, and neurological symptoms (celiac.org).

In my opinion wheat sensitivity is a more difficult intolerance to deal with than milk since it is found in nearly everything in the United States as a refined wheat or whole-grain product. Its wholeness really doesn't matter, though I must admit I think sometimes the whole grain is more reactive than white flour foods, which are less nutritious. People are really attached to bread and a lot of refined wheat confectionary foods (crackers, pastries, pretzels, etc.), which are not only vehicles for sweet-fat calories but may also trigger food intolerance. Interestingly, if you ate a traditional rice-based Asian diet, you would not even think about dairy products and wheat in bread. They wouldn't be in your normal diet. The rice-based Asian diet is a "low allergy" diet by nature.

Why Are Wheat and Dairy Products Addictive?

Wheat, like dairy products, contain opioid compounds: gliado (or gluteo) morphin or exorphins. These are addictive compounds. Gliadin is a fraction of the wheat protein gluten. Exorphins are found in food proteins, while endorphins, the "feel good" neurochemicals, are made within the body. These exorphins, opioid-like peptides (small chains of amino acids), can alter neuron function in the brain. The gliado- and casomorphin (milk opioid) compounds can also trigger inflammation in the gut, making it more permeable (intestinal permeability). This can allow for a variety of components from the intestinal tract to be absorbed and trigger a reaction that results in a systemic complaint, meaning somewhere else in your body (e.g., headache, joint pain, fatigue, etc.).

Why "Food Intolerance" and Not "Food Allergy"?

I choose the term "food intolerance" because there is no single good definition of food allergy that includes all reactions to foods. When most allergists say food allergy, they generally mean an IgE mediated response. This is usually immediate, can be severe or life threatening, and is most commonly diagnosed by RAST testing (blood test) or a skin prick or scratch test. Patients usually know their IgE mediated reactions because they are generally quite obvious. There is a small frequency of this type of food reaction. Subsequently many allergists say the suffering individual does not have food allergies.

Our bodies, though, can react in many different ways to a food. It can be a direct IgE mediated type of response as mentioned; an IgG response (a delayed response to food); immune complexes, which exist in the body for very short periods of time but can be deposited in joint space or other tissues; biochemical reactions like MSG (monosodium glutamate); neurochemical responses to the chemical structure of a substance like aspartame; an enzyme insufficiency such as lactose intolerance where the enzyme is lacking to break down milk sugar; or an enzyme lack (disaccharidase) on the folds of the intestine, resulting in carbohydrate malabsorption in the gut; lectins on foods that may react to one's blood type; absorption of toxic organic acids derived from bacteria and fungus in the gut; the white blood cell, or leukocyte, just reacting to a food; certain foods affecting the autonomic nervous system differently (parasympathetic and sympathetic); and other ways we can react to food.

This is why I use "food intolerance" as a catch-all definition for any reaction to a food instead of using the term "food allergy." This tends to be a less "politically" charged definition!

Testing for Food Intolerance

Testing for food allergy or intolerance is controversial and debatable. When I talk to patients, I tell them there is no one test that can test for all the ways their body reacts to foods. Many tests are not completely accurate; there are many false positives. (A false positive is when the test says there is a reaction when there really isn't.) Though not perfect, a test can still be valuable clinically yet have a significant amount of false positives.

For example, if ten foods showed up on whatever allergy test you take as positive and only three are true reactants, but you eliminate all ten foods, you will still have improvement in some of your symptoms (e.g., headaches, joint pain, gastrointestinal distress, etc.). The key to any food intolerance test is to eliminate the foods that are positive reactors and reintroduce the **most commonly eaten foods first** so you can identify which foods are the most significant offenders. The reactors should be eliminated for one to six months and then reintroduced. Starting with the most commonly eaten foods makes the most sense. I tell patients that if you eat garbanzo beans once a month but you have daily headaches, the garbanzo bean is probably not the major problem food, even if it is a true reactant. Focus on the foods you are eating three or more times per week first for reintroduction.

A very important point is that just because a food doesn't show up on the test doesn't necessarily mean you are not sensitive to it. If you feel bad after eating, it is the food until proven otherwise—positive test or not. Trust how you feel. Write down the food and your symptoms in your diet diary. Eliminate the food. A month later, re-challenge yourself to find out how you feel.

The Basic Elimination Diet (see Appendix A), or what I call the "Poor Person's Food Allergy Test," was designed to eliminate many of the classic allergens such as dairy, wheat, glutinous grains (oat, barley, rye), corn, eggs, yeast, chocolate, tomato, citrus, peanuts, nightshade family (potatoes, tomatoes, eggplant, peppers, etc.), and a few others. This list can be used as a simple shopping list. All you do is fill up your refrigerator and cupboards with these foods in their whole state and eat away for two to four weeks. See how you feel and chart your symptoms on the Diet-Exercise-Symptom Diary (see Educational Handouts at Prescription2000.com). After at least two weeks (preferably one month), add in foods one at a time, a day or so apart, starting with the most frequently eaten. If there is a reaction within twenty-four hours, eliminate the food again, this time for three months, and then try it again. If done right, you may save thousands of dollars not only on allergy testing but on your overall health as well.

Food intolerance can cause, aggravate, be part of, or be the total cause of symptoms that people have been living with for years. I can't tell you how many times I have asked people what they eat for breakfast, lunch, dinner, and snacks, what they drink and crave, and some of those "biggies" come up (dairy, wheat, sugar, etc.). Many times, these patients have gone from doctor to doctor, including specialists, and no one has ever simply asked them what they eat or suggested that food could be a problem. This is so sad and unfortunate. Simply eliminating just one of those foods can sometimes make a profound difference. Remember this: Be willing to look at the foods you commonly eat—those you eat daily or really like—if you have a chronic problem. Then try to eliminate it (two to four of them) for one month. Many of you will be surprised. If done right, food elimination is the single most powerful tool in medicine.

Chapter 12

"ALLERGIC LOAD" AND DETOXIFICATION

Your "Allergic Load"

The term "allergic load" simply means the total challenge to your immune system and metabolism that comes from the foods you consume; the environment that you touch and breathe; the state of your internal biochemistry, especially your liver and gastrointestinal functioning; and the mind-body perception of your life. All these things can trigger neuroendocrine and immunologic pathways that cause abnormal or hyper responses to the environment. Together, all of these components create your "allergic load" and can tip your allergic "teeter totter" toward manifesting significant symptoms. One component alone may not do it.

There is a mind-body connection with allergy or hypersensitivity. If you are chronically in a mental state of fight or flight, then you are putting out more cortisol, an anti-inflammatory hormone. With time, this chronic fight-or-flight lifestyle may result in the inability to put out cortisol at appropriate periods of stress or allergy exposure, and then you have more manifestation of the symptoms.

Seasonal Allergies and Your Allergic Load

Seasonal allergies can be reduced by paying attention to your allergic load. I have seen this scenario every year for more than two decades. If people go on a low-allergy, whole-food diet; take some anti-inflammatory nutrients such as vitamins C, E, and D, quercetin, fish oil, and flax and/or primrose oil; normalize gut function by either replacement of the good bacteria or killing of abnormal pathogens (yeast, overgrowth of bacteria, parasites); clean up their home environment, especially their bedroom; and flush their sinuses several times per day, what they will find with the next allergy season is that their seasonal allergies are much lessened.

All types of allergies are interconnected. If you reduce food sensitivities, you generally have less inhalant allergies when the next season comes around and vice versa. So when people get worried about the upcoming "allergy season," I really try to get them to look at the bigger picture of their food intake, home environment, and gut function, in addition to addressing their upcoming inhalant allergy concerns.

Controlling Your Immediate Environment and Allergic Load

Environmental control is critically important. One must work from the bedroom, through the home, to the work environment, and to the world. A handout I use for patients, "How to Allergy-Proof a Bedroom," shows an optimal environmentally clean bedroom and is available at NationalAllergySupply.com. There are many very simple things that can be done to reduce the insults you receive in the place most people spend most of their time—the bedroom:

- Use blinds or shades (no hanging drapes)
- Low-pile carpets or hardwood floors
- Mattress and pillowcase covers
- HEPA air filters and humidifiers in the bedroom
- Filters for the vents
- *No* stuffed animals or dolls on the bed
- ***No* pets** in the bedroom! ***No* pets** on the bed!

If you clean the bedroom as described and you still wake up in the morning congested, look outside your window for some kind of pollen. Also, try to remember the last time you spilled something on the floor. Look for mold. Just pull up the carpet and peek. The other thing to consider is what you ate the night before or every evening. That nightly bowl of ice cream, glass of milk, hunk of cheese, grilled-cheese sandwich, piece of pie or cookies, or alcoholic beverage may be the cause of your brain fog, snotty nose, productive cough, or crusty eyes the following morning. Many times, it is that simple. Now if you add the late-night snack to the dusty bedroom and the pet sleeping next to you, you may not only be a "mess" in the morning but you may start off very fatigued as well. Any of you seeing yourself yet?

Aside from cleaning up the bedroom and not eating offending food the night before, one of the simplest things that can dramatically improve your morning symptoms and health is a *facial rinse* or *sinus flush* morning and evening.

To do the facial rinse, plug the sink, fill it with hot water (test it with your chin; **don't burn yourself!**), pour in two or three teaspoons of salt, and immerse your face completely in the hot water. Hold it for five seconds, and then lift your face from the water and blow your nose. Repeat this sequence four or five times over the next few minutes. This simple technique can help clear out your sinuses, reducing your annoying symptoms almost immediately. This simple technique also helps to reduce your allergic load.

The "sister" technique to this is the sinus flush. This is usually done while in the shower. Get a blue bulb syringe. Cut the tip so it fits snuggly up your nose. Put one to two teaspoons of salt into a bowl of *lukewarm* water. Suck up the water into the syringe and, while you are in the shower, stick the syringe up one nostril. Tilt your head forward and squirt it up your nose. It's kind of messy and might sting a bit, but it works. Together these two techniques, if done consistently, can reduce nasal congestion, sometimes dramatically. Especially when done with food elimination the night before.

There are a variety of other "sinus flush" devices that you can commercially buy as well. Usually I will just cup my hands underneath my nose in the shower to catch the water and snort it. Occasionally I get that sting, but it helps. It's the "lazy man's" sinus flush. It doesn't sound impressive, but it works for a busy guy like me.

An additional "allergy trick" is to take one-quarter to one teaspoon of vitamin C powder (usually this equals 1,000 to 4,000 mg) just before bed and as soon as you wake up. Start with one-quarter teaspoon at night and in the morning. As long as your stools don't get loose, you can increase up to a full or rounded teaspoon at night and in the morning. This little pearl obviously works better if you have a clean bedroom environment, have flushed your sinuses, and haven't eaten offending foods the night before. But it will help you feel better in the morning even if you haven't done those common sense things to reduce your morning allergy symptoms. Vitamin C taken orally has been shown to reduce histamine levels, and one of its highest concentrations in the body is the adrenal glands, which are the almond-size glands on our kidneys that put out anti-inflammatory hormones.[1]

Remember:
"Allergic load" equals food *plus* environment *plus* internal systems (adrenal, liver, gut) *plus* mind-body.

How Does Our Gut Affect Allergy Development?

The internal milieu of the body is critical to the outward manifestation of allergy. There are more micro-organisms (bacteria) in the gut than there are cells in our bodies. If you compacted all the micro-organisms in the gut, they would weigh approximately the same as your liver. These micro-organisms do many things, including affecting your overall immune system by affecting your gut immune system. Healthy gut bacteria are critical for reducing your allergic load. If you enhance the normal bacterial flora with such probiotics as Lactobacillus, Bifidobacterium, or Lactobacillus *rhamnosus*, you can make sure other competitive organisms, bacteria, and fungi do not grow in excess, causing inflammation of the gastrointestinal mucosa and increasing the risk of allergy and food intolerance.

It has been shown that probiotics such as Lactobacillus *rhamnosus*, when given to mothers during pregnancy and/or lactation, and to the infants as soon as they are born, result in fewer allergies (atopy) later on in life.[2]

You will see the term "probiotic" all over the Internet and in medical journals. These organisms are the subject of intense research and may even be valuable in the critical care setting in hospitals by reducing infection and sepsis and length of hospital stay.[3]

At an international meeting on probiotics in Córdoba, Argentina, in October 2001, this working definition for probiotics was agreed upon for the meeting: "Live microorganisms which when administered in adequate amounts confer a health benefit on the host," but limited the scope of the discussion to "Live microorganisms which when consumed in adequate amounts as part of food confer a health benefit on the host." [4]

Good digestion is very important in reducing food intolerance. The smaller the fragments of food absorbed through the gut, the less likely they may trigger a reaction or be recognized by your immune system as a foreign substance. If the gut wall is inflamed enough to cause increased intestinal permeability (bigger sieve-like holes in the gut wall), then bigger than normal molecules could be absorbed, triggering even more and greater food reactions anywhere in the body.[5]

"Intestinal permeability" is a term you should remember. It means damage to the bowel lining, caused by medications, toxins, poor diet, food intolerance, parasites, fungus, bacterial overgrowth, or infection. Intestinal permeability can lead to toxins, microbes, undigested food, waste, or larger than normal macromolecules being absorbed and causing a reaction locally or elsewhere in the body.[6]

Change in intestinal permeability is one variable why symptoms to foods can change from allergy test to allergy test or with time. If your intestinal permeability is reduced, you will have smaller sieve-like holes in your gut and less uptake of foreign material through the gut wall that might trigger a reaction some-where else in your body. This is one of the main reasons why, to help many chronically ill patients with multiple complaints, you not only evaluate them for food intolerance but also for "bugs" and abnormal bacteria in the gut. Using probiotics and treating any gut infections can improve intestinal permeability and reduce the allergic load and many bodily complaints that are far away from the gut (e.g., headaches, joint pain, sinus congestion, asthma, etc.).

Toxic Metals and Allergic Load

Metal toxicity is a very controversial area. It can definitely aggravate one's allergic load. The question is not whether *acute exposure* to toxic metals (lead, cadmium, mercury, arsenic, aluminum, nickel, manganese, selenium, etc.) is harmful, because it obviously is. The question is whether low-level *chronic exposure* to these metals can cause chronic health problems. I believe the answer is yes, but it is not so easy to quantify and treat.

In the 1970s, the great Herbert Needleman, MD, a pediatrician from the University of Pittsburgh, discovered elevated lead in the teeth of children and correlated this level with lowered cognitive function/IQ in poorer children, and then, to his surprise, in well-to-do children as well. This led Dr. Needleman on an odyssey that eventually directed him to take on big oil in getting lead out of gasoline after showing that nationwide lead exposure correlated with criminal behavior and that elevated lead in the blood correlated with lowered IQ levels.[7]

At our clinic, we measure toxic metals with a six-hour urine collection after an intravenous chelation challenge. If you do a pre- and post-urine challenge for toxic metals, most of the time, you see no metals in the urine before the chelation challenge. If you do find metal elevation in the pre-challenge urine, it is likely to be an acute exposure. While we virtually never see elevated metals pre-challenge, we frequently see patients who have some type of significantly elevated metals post-chelation challenge. What we are looking for is a five-fold or more increase over the normal range.

Now comes the hard part: what to do about heavy metals—if anything. While logic says to remove them, we don't yet know all the ramifications of removing these excessive metals. We do know that these metals can cause problems with different metabolic pathways and result in some serious complications of human health. The problem lies in knowing what level is toxic and really harmful when these metals are stored in your body. Questions to be answered are: What happens when you take these metals out of the body? What problems do they cause on the way out? What are the best and safest chelating agents? Where are all these metals coming from? When stored in body tissues, nerves, bone, and organs for years, what damage are they really doing?

We need more research in this area. There is no question there is an excess body burden of toxic metals in many people by this type of testing. Physicians who approach this complex problem can be found at the American College for Advancement in Medicine (ACAM.org).

Detoxing: What Does It Mean?

One of my pet peeves is the way the word "detoxing" is thrown around in alternative medicine. People make it sound as if they actually know what is occurring in the body when they do their particular program; that the way their product improves these incredible pathways of detoxification in the body (liver, skin, bowels, respiration, etc.) is a proven thing. The truth is that most people who talk about detoxing have no idea about the complicated biochemistry of detoxification. What they do know is that when they put others on a very simple diet with some type of detox product, many symptoms improve. The promoters of the detox products imply their product is doing the detoxing so you have something to buy from them. The truth is that most of the time a very simple and elemental diet is the magic (my opinion). That doesn't mean fiber-type supplements, probiotics, antioxidants, phytochemicals and nutrients that stimulate liver function don't benefit detoxification, because they can. Still, the biggest part is what people eat (or, truthfully, what they *don't* eat) during the detox program.

Skin is one of the greatest detoxification organs. Sweating by any measure, whether in a far infrared sauna, regular saunas (wet or dry), or exercise, is a very important way to eliminate chronic toxins. Just sweating on a regular basis is important. So hard exercise is not only good for your vascular system, but it also helps detoxify your body at the same time and costs nothing! I recently asked a lecturer at a conference who was speaking on heavy metal detoxification what he thought about far infrared saunas versus other types of saunas. He felt that sweating was sweating. It's all good for reducing the toxin load no matter how you do it. Just sweat!

Another very important way to detoxify is to have regular, bulky bowel movements, several times per day. High-fiber, plant-based diets provide the bulk for easy elimination and the antioxidants, vitamins, minerals, and phytochemicals to support any detoxification process.

When you go on a detoxification program, you are getting off foods you commonly eat and resting your immune system and biochemistry from immune challenge from them. Fasting is the extreme example of this. That is mainly why people improve, in my opinion. In addition, most cleansing diets are some kind of simple, vegetable-based diets. These diets tend to be low in common allergens and high in nutrient-rich plant foods (like greens), which help provide antioxidant compounds that aid in detoxification and protection of body tissue. So the "magic" of these so-called detox programs is many times just that: getting you on an elemental diet that rests the immune system, and many times these diets are antioxidant-rich plant foods low in total calories.

Simple "Detox Program" (one to three weeks)

- Eat as many fruit and vegetables as you want (raw, steamed, lightly stir-fried in vegetable broth or water) or vegetable soups from the BED List (Appendix A).

- Make half your food green vegetables, preferably leafy.
- Drink six to eight 8-ounce glasses of water per day at least. Mineral water, decaffeinated green or black teas, or herbal teas are acceptable.
- Take vitamin C (2,000 mg/d), and a general multivitamin/minerals/d. (If you experience any muscle cramps, take calcium [400–800 mg/d] and magnesium [400–800 mg/d] with food.)
- Keep a diet-symptom diary of food intake and how you feel.
- Do *gentle* movement, such as walking and stretching, daily. Do not push yourself.
- Reintroduce food slowly with whole grains, nuts or seeds, and beans in addition to your vegetables and fruit for two weeks and then free-range animal foods, if desired, though this is not recommended. Avoid dairy for at least two more weeks (preferably don't reintroduce at all).
- Keep using your diet-exercise-symptom diary when adding in new foods.

There are many variations of this. Some might add a small amount of protein or "good" carbohydrate. On this type of simple diet, you can't be doing a lot of physical activity. It's a "gentle" time. You should check with your doctor first, especially if you are on multiple medications since the sudden weight loss could result in over-medication symptoms.

Fasting: The Ultimate Detox and Anti-Inflammatory Diet

Recently I had the pleasure of interviewing Dr. Alan Goldhamer, founder and director of TrueNorth Health in Santa Rosa, California (healthpromoting.com), where therapeutic fasting is done under medical supervision for common and severe medical conditions. Dr. Goldhamer and his colleagues have supervised more than seven thousand water fasts. Fasting, when done appropriately, is one of the most powerful tools in medicine for healing. Fasting, by definition, is just with water. At TrueNorth, juice and water fasts are done from several days up to forty days. If you haven't been able to gain control of your health or have a chronic illness, a medically supervised fast may be a life changer.[8]

Part III:
The Program

TRIAD Wellness Program

The **TRIAD Wellness Program** acknowledges that there are three integrated disciplines and areas of focus that contribute to our overall wellness: Diet, Exercise, and the Mind-Body. For each of these key areas of health, there are three simple practices to keep you functioning at your healthiest. All together, these result in the *9 Simple Steps to Optimal Health*. However you choose to remember these daily health habits is up to you. I just hope you not only remember them easily but also practice them daily. I know if you do you will get results, and steadily (sometimes quickly) you will become the director of your health journey, which is my wish for you.

The next part of this book breaks down each of these three phases of the **TRIAD Wellness Program**: The TRIAD Diet Program (Steps 1, 2, and 3), the TRIAD Exercise Program (Steps 4, 5, and 6), and the TRIAD Mind-Body Program (Steps 7, 8, and 9). I will go over the background of each of these phases and why they are so important to your overall health; what each step means; and how to implement these steps in the busy, modern world.

It is hard for many to accept that good health can really be achieved by practicing daily, very simple and non-complicated principles as the *9 Simple Steps to Optimal Health*, but it's true. Like anyone who is a master at their craft, more often than not they will tell you that it's the basic fundamentals they do day in and day out that allow them to complete amazing tasks at a higher level. It's the daily practice of these basics, those *9 Simple Steps to Optimal Health,* that create the magic of good health.

I hope to convince you through the next part of this book that these steps are not only logical but also doable despite your busy lifestyle. I hope I can convince you and motivate you enough that you will give these principles at least a three-month trial.

The **TRIAD Wellness Program** is a very practical system to achieve real healthcare reform and real health security in a very busy world as individuals, a country, and the world. All you have to do is just follow the steps. *It is that simple!*

Chapter 13

THE TRIAD DIET PROGRAM

Steps 1, 2, and 3 of the *9 Simple Steps to Optimal Health*

- **(Step 1) EAT whole**, unprocessed **foods** (90 percent or more as plant foods, if not all plant foods).
- **(Step 2) EAT** at least **half** your food intake as **vegetables**.
- **(Step 3) ELIMINATE** all **dairy products** or eat from the Basic Elimination Diet (BED) for at least one month.

Most of the time, you can identify w*hole foods* just by looking at them—because they are just that: *whole food* in front of you.

In general, if something is in a package, box, or can, choose the one with the least amount of things added to it. You just want the food. Take canned beans, for example. I look at the label and try to make sure there is no added sugar. (I don't worry as much about salt since I sweat a lot and am very active, but in general, I tell patients to go salt-free and make sure there are no additives.) Just the beans are what you want. And now it's easy to get even canned organic beans at stores like Trader Joe's, Whole Foods Market, and natural food co-ops. These canned goods have fewer additives.

Of course you'll want to eat more than just beans, so here are my guidelines for a good diet—which are really very similar to those recommended by the WHO and Unified Dietary Guidelines:

- Greater than 90 percent of your food intake should be *unrefined* plant foods. **(Step 1)**
- Eat vegetables, especially green leafy vegetables, fruit, beans, nuts, and seeds in their whole state and as close to how they came out of the ground.

- Consume whole or sprouted grains only.
- Do not eat refined carbohydrates.
- Do not eat refined fats, hydrogenated vegetable oils, or trans-fatty acids.
- You can use raw nuts and seeds, ground flaxseed in small amounts (two-three tablespoons per day), unless you are very active and need to maintain or put on weight, then you can consume more. Use cold-pressed extra-virgin olive oil and canola oil sparingly. Cook more with vegetable (organic) broth than oil.
- **Optional (not necessary):** Consume small amounts of eggs, game, fish, poultry, and meat (free-ranged, grass-fed, antibiotic-and hormone-free, or wild game if animal foods are eaten).
- Drink at least five to six glasses of water per day.
- At least half your food intake should be vegetables. **(Step 2)**
- No dairy products! (If you must, do at least a one-month trial off ALL dairy products completely.) Or better yet eat from the Basic Elimination Diet (Appendix A) list for four weeks while applying Steps 1 and 2. **(Step 3)**

That is it—really! A good diet is that simple. There are no complex rules or fancy gimmicks. Just eat the food groups listed above in their most *whole state*. And for most people, especially if your weight is normalized, you don't have to worry about portions. Eating these types of whole foods until you are satisfied is all you have to do.

The "Pizza Platter" Test for a Good Diet

Imagine that you take all the food you eat all day long and dump it on an *extra extra* large pizza platter on your living room floor. If you look down on it at the end of the day, ideally 100 percent of it should be whole, unprocessed foods. Ninety percent or more of that should be whole, unrefined plant foods. Specifically, one-half or more of the pizza platter should be vegetables, half of which (or one-quarter of the platter) should be green, leafy vegetables.

The other half of the platter can be a combination of fruit, beans, whole grains, nuts and seeds, and, if you must (optional but not recommended), small amounts of fish, eggs, poultry, and meat. That's what I call the "pizza platter" test of how to estimate a good diet. As far as I'm concerned, it beats the heck out of thinking about serving sizes!

It's Simple: Surround Yourself with Whole Foods Only!

If you eat whole foods, shop for whole foods, and only have whole foods in your cupboards and refrigerator, then you do not have to worry about added sweet-fat calories (added sweeteners, fats, refined grains). If you are eating minimal or no animal foods then you do not have to worry about excess calories, protein, saturated fat, cholesterol, and other fats from the meat, especially non-grass-fed animals. Remember our Paleolithic lesson: Meat is an energy-dense food. It helped man survive because wild game was a good protein, fat, and calorie source. We don't need as much energy-dense foods in this day and age of modern transportation and easy access to calories, especially fat-laden, grain-fed meats from sedentary animals that were given hormones and antibiotics! We need nutrient-dense foods with low caloric density (generally). Those are the unrefined plant foods.

Nutrient Density: Why Is This So Important?

I have mentioned the term "nutrient density" many times in this book. It is one of the most important concepts in basic health and nutrition. Just for the sake of demonstration, set down this book for a moment and hold out both of your hands, arms spread and palms up. Imagine you're holding in your right hand one hundred calories of white sugar and in your left hand one hundred calories of beans or broccoli. Which is better for you?

I'll bet you said that the beans or broccoli are better for you—and you're right. But do you know why? The reason is that while the white sugar in your right hand has calories that your cells need to function, it contains no vitamins, minerals, fiber, and phytonutrients to help protect you against chronic disease and to metabolize those calories. It also spikes blood sugar and insulin levels that can have adverse health consequences if repetitively consumed. Beans on the other hand, have added fiber, complex carbohydrates, protein, and good fats, and they regulate your blood sugar well. Broccoli is high in protein, fiber, and in minerals like calcium and magnesium. Broccoli also contains powerful antioxidant and detoxifying compounds, such as sulforaphane, that protect against cancer and help metabolize estrogen to a less-risky form. So the broccoli and beans are more "nutrient-dense" than white sugar even though they have the same amount of calories as the sugar—and better for you!

Joel Fuhrman, MD (drfuhrman.com), who wrote what I consider to be one of the best health books ever, *Eat To Live* (2011), and also a two-volume series of excellent diet-nutrition books called *Eat For Health* (2008), takes the concept of nutrient density and gives it a different name. He calls it the **Health Equation: H = N/C (nutrients/calories)**. He states, "Your health is predicted by your nutrient intake divided by your intake of calories."[1]

In this equation, true health is dependent on the nutrient-per-calorie density of the diet. I could not agree more. In his books, he actually evaluates the nutrient density, or "health equation," of many different foods and food groups and ranks them from high nutrient-per-calorie density to low. He calls this ranking an ANDI score—Aggregate Nutrient Density Index. It is not surprising that the foods from highest to lowest nutrient density are the green leafy vegetables; then solid greens; all raw vegetables; non-starchy cooked vegetables; fresh fruit; beans/legumes; cooked starchy vegetables; whole grains; raw nuts or seeds; then low-fat animal foods; and, lastly, refined grains; full-fat dairy products; cheeses; refined oils; and sweets.[2]

What Is Caloric Density?

"Caloric density" (CD) means how many calories you have per weight/mass of food. It is kind of like the "sister" of nutrient density. Using them together—consuming foods with high nutrient density and low caloric density—is the prescription for a healthy diet that we can eat a lot of and still stay lean and healthy. Usually caloric density is calculated to be the amount of calories contained in one gram of a given food (calories/grams = CD).[3] So, to find the CD of a food, look at the serving size on the label. Put the calories of the serving size over the weight in grams of the serving size. Then you can calculate the caloric density.

- Very Low Caloric Density = 0.0 to 0.7
- Low to Moderate Caloric Density = 0.8 to 1.5
- Moderate to High Caloric Density = 1.6 to 3.0
- Very High Caloric Density = 3.1 and up

Let's see how this translates to the foods we actually eat:[4]

- A whole apple contains 72 calories and weighs 132 grams. Therefore the caloric density of one apple is .57 (78 cal/138 g), which is a very low caloric density, so you can virtually eat all the apples you want.
- A plain enriched bagel is 71 grams and 182 calories. Its caloric density is 2.56 (182 cal/71 g). This has a moderate to high caloric density. You want to watch your portion size.
- One ounce of almonds (24 almonds) is 28.35 grams or 163 calories, which provides a caloric density of 5.6 (163 cal/28.35 g). This is very high, so you want to eat this amount sparingly.
- A three-ounce piece of lean, fat-trimmed, top sirloin steak that has been broiled has a caloric density of 1.91 (163 cal/85 gm), which is in the moderate to high range. That means you need to watch your portion size.
- One tablespoon of olive oil is 13.5 grams and 119 calories. This small amount of oil has a caloric density of 8.8 (119 cal/13.5 g), which is very high. You want to eat this amount sparingly.

Reducing Caloric Density

You can reduce the CD of your diet by understanding a couple of principles. If most of your diet is whole fruit and vegetables, then you have a great start to reducing CD. You can generally eat as much of these two food groups as you want. Be cautious about eating too much dried fruit because it takes the water content out and makes it a high-calorie-dense food (concentrates the sugar as well). Remember: Foods high in water content (including fruit, soups, and cooked grains) and fiber dilute calories and naturally reduce the CD. They also generally happen to be very high in nutrient density as well.

Cooked whole grains, beans, and potatoes in their skin are in the moderate caloric density range, along with lean fish and poultry. I would choose these plant foods over the animal foods in moderation because they have fiber and provide more bulk in the stomach, and they contain more micronutrients. If you take this same amount of cooked grain and make it into bread with whole or refined grain flour, you increase the CD significantly (up to seven times).[5]

Even though I have been encouraging whole, sprouted grain breads as more nutritious and health promoting than refined flour breads, the truth is that one slice of bread, whether from refined wheat flour or whole or sprouted wheat, is essentially the same in caloric density. Bread is still a moderately high calorically dense food, and you need to watch how many servings of bread products you eat (in fact, the CD of a slice of the sprouted whole grain bread I eat was 2.64, and a slice of pure white sandwich bread in the local grocery store was 2.5). Generally, but not always, as the fiber content of the bread increases, the CD goes down, refined or whole grain. This is one reason people recommend going off all bread on a weight loss regime. But—here is a big **IF**!—if you are eating a whole- or sprouted-grain versus a refined-grain bread, you will eat less of the whole-grain bread because it will provide more bulk from its higher fiber content and is more nutrient dense. So you will feel fuller, and the whole grain will stabilize your blood sugar better so you won't crave and eat more of it to be satisfied. The whole-grain slice of bread is also more nutrient dense, which helps reduce hunger, so it is still a much better choice than refined-flour bread, even though the caloric densities are similar.

I have done this experiment personally many times. While shopping, I'll throw a medium-size loaf of fresh sourdough in my shopping cart. By the time I get to the checkout counter, it's gone. If that were my whole grain, sprouted grain loaf of bread, I might be able to consume one piece, maybe two, and be full. Watch the amount of baked grain products (refined or not) that you eat if you are trying to control your weight, and only buy whole or sprouted grain products to have in your home.

Check the CD of Your Snack Food

I am generally not a label reader and don't really want you to spend lots of time reading labels. I just want you to see whole food and put it in your shopping cart, refrigerator, and cupboards. But here is a worthwhile exercise. Take your favorite four or five snack foods and look at their CD. Look at the serving size. Take the total calories and divide it by the grams of a serving size. You may be very surprised at the high CD of your snack foods.

As I am writing this book, my refrigerator and cupboards are literally ten feet behind me. So I get up and stress eat from anxiousness on some aspect of the editing, researching, or writing of this book. After I get bored with the whole fruit in my refrigerator, I might eat a slice of sprouted rye bread (CD 2.64), tamari roasted almonds (CD 5.66), plain dried mango slices (CD 3.15), or splurge on that "low carb," gluten-free, no trans-fat, no sugar added dark chocolate with almond bar (CD 4.4).

As you can see, after becoming bored with my fruit and veggies those other snack foods are almost always high in CD. I am well aware of that and watch it. If I was struggling with my weight and did not understand that even these relatively whole-looking foods would be making my weight loss very difficult, I could become frustrated. It is very educational and can be a fun experience to get a pad of paper and take ten of your favorite foods and find their CD.

This may help you significantly control the types and amounts of foods you consume. Have fun with it. Understanding and applying the concept of CD could be a life saver!

The Okinawa Diet™ Caloric Density Pyramid

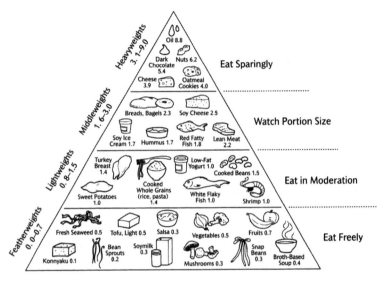

With permission. Okinawa Diet Plan. website: www.okinawa-diet.com
http://okinawaprogram.com/okinawa_diet/caloric_density_pyramid.html

A Word about "Volumetrics"

The *Volumetrics Eating Plan* (Volumetricseatingplan.com), written by Dr. Barbara J. Rolls, focuses on creating satiety by eating foods that create the feeling of fullness while at the same time consuming fewer calories.[6] Foods with higher water content have fewer calories, such as fruit, vegetables, and soups. Dr. Rolls' research has shown that most people eat the same weight or volume of foods at meals. Therefore, if one eats as we have been discussing, high nutrient-dense, low calorie-dense foods, which take up volume either by water content or fiber, a feeling of fullness is more likely with improved nutrient intake while losing weight. Energy density, which is the same as caloric density, is a concept she uses as well. Most overweight Americans should try to eat low, energy-dense foods that are higher in bulk (volume).

This concept of volumetrics is simply demonstrated in the following illustration of "three stomachs" taken from Dr. Joel Fuhrman's excellent book, *Eat to Live* (2011).[7] Eating greater amounts of unrefined plant foods that provide more bulk but fewer calories is the natural way to satiety and maintaining optimal weight.

MORE BULK MEANS FEWER CALORIES

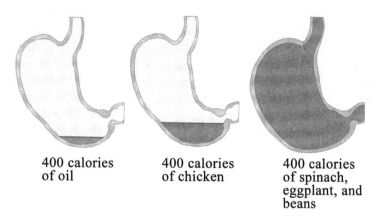

400 calories of oil	400 calories of chicken	400 calories of spinach, eggplant, and beans

With permission from Joel Fuhrman, MD. Drfuhrman.com

Hara Hachi Bu

In Okinawa, they have a saying, "*hara hachi bu,*" which means something like "eat until you are 80 percent full (or eight parts full)." Once Okinawan elders initially feel satisfied, they do not continue eating until they really feel full. This practice is hard for us in the West because we have so much food available. The Okinawan elders do this naturally, along with naturally consuming lower calorie-dense, high nutrient-dense foods.

Vegetables

The only way you can mess up vegetables is by not eating them at all. Even if you cook the life out of them, they will still be an improvement if they replace excess calories from meat, cheeses, added sweeteners, fats and oils, and refined grains. I have no problem with frozen vegetables. Obviously it would be best if you could eat organically grown foods from your backyard, picked fifteen minutes before you eat them, but first, just eat vegetables—and lots of them! Eat them raw, steamed, lightly sautéed, stir fried, whatever. Try cooking with organic vegetable broth (my new cooking essential) instead of oils or animal broth. It works great to make bland things tasteful. Generally speaking, if the vegetable still has some brightness in its color after you have lightly cooked it, then you have done a good job. Low sodium organic vegetable broths are available for those with blood pressure or sodium effected health problems.

Half your daily food intake at least should be vegetables. Half of that intake of vegetables, or one-quarter of your daily total, should be the most nutrient-dense of all whole foods: green, leafy vegetables (kale, chard, spinach, mustard greens, arugula, collards, romaine lettuce—any kind of green leafy that you can get down). Greens *per calorie* have as much protein as a steak. When you think about it, it is really obvious. Where do you think all the green leafy vegetation and grass-consuming large animals (elephants, rhinos, giraffes, hippos, gorillas, etc.) get their protein (and strong bones)? They don't eat each other. They don't drink milk or eat cheese. They don't eat fish. It's obvious. By consuming massive amounts of green, usually leafy, plant foods!

Fruit

Like vegetables, calories from whole fruit replace those from refined, processed, empty-calorie foods. Just be sure to eat the whole fruit, fresh or frozen, as close to its coming off the tree, bush, or vine as you can. Eat color and make sure you throw in some berries daily (purple, blue, red, containing anthocyanidins) that can help protect your eyes from macular degeneration and keep them healthy, among other body benefits. Fruit is loaded with antioxidants and phytochemicals that protect your body and help direct your genes in the way we evolved. The whole fruit is better than the sauce or puree, which is better than the freshly made juice, which is better than the reconstituted juice, and so on.

People bash fruit a lot because of the sugar content, but this is way overblown. Fructose (monosaccharide), which is fruit sugar, is metabolized differently and slower than glucose or sucrose (table sugar). Fructose must go to the liver first to be metabolized. Secondly, when you eat the whole fruit, you are diluting the calories in that fruit with water and fiber. It will be more slowly absorbed than the fresh-squeezed juice or if it was pureed into a sauce (e.g., applesauce). Eating a whole fruit is not at all like taking a gulp of high fructose corn syrup, which is a concentrated mixture of glucose and fructose without any fiber or phytonutrients.

A Note about Fruit and Vegetable Concentrates

It is very popular now to consume one or several different fruit or vegetable extracts, juices, or concentrates (sold usually in a multilevel marketing structure) or the whole "green drinks" in powder form. In general, I don't have a problem with patients picking out one or two they like, feel better with, or seem to resonate with on some level. But—here is my *big but!*—don't replace whole fruit and vegetables with any drink or supplement. Just don't do it! This mentality is flawed. Eat a wide variety of whole fruit and vegetables, and *supplement* a good whole-food diet with your juice/ vegetable drink *du jour* if you want.

Beans

Beans are a fabulous food because they are rich in protein, slow-release carbohydrates, fiber, and vitamins and minerals. They are great for diabetics, weight loss, and heart disease patients provided they don't come with a bunch of extra calories from fat, meats, and cheeses added to them.

Aside from just eating the whole bean or putting them in soups, they can also be mashed into spreads that are much tastier and better for you than those creamy, white junk sauces that are often served in the middle of an otherwise healthy vegetable platter (drives me crazy!). The next time you throw a party or attend a potluck or sporting event, replace the usual high-calorie and fat-laden creamy dip with a nice bean spread (white, black, garbanzo, pinto, etc). Your friends will be so distracted by how good it tastes that they won't even realize you've tricked them into eating something that is great for their health! The simplest version of a healthy bean spread can be made by taking your favorite bean (organic if possible) and blending it up in a food processor, then adding garlic, herbs, and lemon or lime juice to taste. It's that simple.

Another interesting and positive aspect of beans: not only are they a great blood sugar food, but they also help us to lose weight or maintain it. When you eat beans, a large percentage—approximately 30 percent of the carbohydrates in the bean—doesn't get absorbed into the bloodstream or broken down by the body. It goes into the colon, and the bacteria in the colon break it down and produce short-chain fatty acids. Not only are these fatty acids good for the colon cells but they act as a fuel for the liver to cause more oxidation of fat by the body, which causes us to lose more weight.[8]

No matter the form in which they are served, beans are unfortunately underutilized because initially they tend to give people gas or some other G.I. complaint. Soaking the beans overnight, rinsing them, and then cooking them helps to mitigate these unpleasant effects. Eating beans regularly over one to two months will also help get your gastrointestinal flora adjusted. If you have problems cut your daily consumption of beans in half until your distressing symptoms are gone, then gradually increase your dose of beans to a half or one cup per day. This is a way to mitigate the digestive complaints from beans until your G.I. flora changes. When possible, organic and non-GMO beans are best.

Nuts and Seeds

Most studies on health have involved nuts but not seeds. Yet both (in their whole, raw state—not roasted or salted) have non-oxidized essential fatty acids, vitamins and minerals, fiber, lignans, plant sterols, and protein. These are healthful food components. With respect to cardiovascular health, when replacing calories from the diet, especially meat calories, and not adding additional calories, nuts and seeds have been shown to reduce cholesterol and the incidence of cardiovascular disease and heart attacks.

In the "Nurses' Health Study," women who consumed nuts greater than five times per week had about a 35 percent lower risk of coronary heart disease; 39 percent reduction of fatal coronary heart disease; and a 32 percent reduction in non-fatal heart attacks than those women who rarely ate nuts.[9] In the "Physicians Health Study," men who rarely or never consumed nuts compared to those who consumed nuts two or more times per week had reduced risks of sudden cardiac death of 47 percent and total coronary heart disease death of 30 percent.[10] In a pooled analysis of four U.S. epidemiological studies, those in the highest intake group for nut consumption had an approximately 35 percent reduced risk of coronary heart disease incidence.[11] These are people who weren't eating a whole-food diet. They were just eating an American diet and some of them had nuts and seeds and some of them didn't. And because of that one change, they had a 40 percent or more reduction in sudden cardiac death.

A recent review of nut consumption and chronic disease showed a consistent association between nut consumption and a reduced risk of coronary heart disease; reduced risk of diabetes mellitus among women; and a protective benefit of frequent nut consumption on gallstone diseases in both sexes. Long-term nut consumption is also linked with lower body weight and lower risk of obesity and weight gain.[12]

The main cautions I offer when eating nuts and seeds are these: First, since they contain fat calories, which have nine calories per gram of fat (compared to four calories from carbohydrates or protein), be cautious when eating nuts and seeds while trying to lose weight. There is evidence, though, that having some fat while on a weight loss program may protect against gallstones and help with fat-soluble vitamin absorption. Two or three tablespoons of ground flaxseed per day or a small handful of raw nuts on a weight loss regimen is probably a good thing. Second, roasted nuts can come with oxidized oil from the heat. So eat them raw most of the time. Third, pay attention to food intolerance. Some nuts can be allergy producing. Fourth, don't eat salt-laden nuts. Overall nuts are a super-food, a wonderful source of protein, fiber, vitamin E, and fatty acids that appear to protect against the number one killer—heart disease—when eaten in moderation.

Whole or Sprouted Grains

Whole or sprouted grains have more fiber, vitamins, minerals, fatty acids, and protein, and a more even release of blood sugar than refined grains. Sprouting is a soaking process of the whole grain kernel that occurs until germination and a small sprout slightly extrudes from the kernel. The sprouted grains are then ground up. Some believe sprouting creates a more easily digestible form of grain, with increased bioavailability of key nutrients and breaking down of lectins to make the grain less sensitizing. Sprouted grains are growing in popularity, but I know of no research that clearly shows they have a higher nutrient content or are less sensitizing than whole grains. When sprouting some of the starches turn to sugars—similar to what occurs during fermentation of grains in the traditional production of sourdough breads. Thus, calories and nutrient content should not be affected. Sprouted grains are generally considered whole grains by most experts. That said, if you think you are sensitive to a grain, try a sprouted version for a month and see if you feel better. I am all for clinical experience, whether I can explain it or not.

"Good" Oils?

Extra-virgin olive oil is rich in monounsaturated fatty acids and phenolic antioxidant compounds. It is believed to be cardioprotective and a good source of stable monounsaturated fatty acid. The more dark green and pungent the extra-virgin olive oil, the greater the concentration of antioxidant phenolic compounds. Canola oil is rich in oleic acid (monounsaturated fatty acid) and to a lesser extent, the omega-3 fatty acid, alpha-linolenic acid (ALA). Ground flaxseeds are rich in ALA, the precursor to the popular eicosapentaenoic acid (EPA) and docosahexaenoic acid (DHA) from fish oil (originally from algae). ALA has anti-inflammatory properties in its own right. It is debatable in humans how well ALA gets converted to EPA and DHA to have cardioprotective and neuroprotective properties.

Compare these to the "bad" oils, which include refined fats, hydrogenated vegetable oils, or trans-fatty acids. Aside from being calorie-dense foods and having more than twice the calories as carbohydrates and proteins (nine calories versus four calories per gram), trans-fatty acids get incorporated into the fatty cell membrane and can alter cell-to-cell communication, causing cellular dysfunction. Trans-fatty acids increase cholesterol levels and cardiovascular risk. Refined oils are exposed to more heat and can have more lipid peroxides (oxidized fat), which can damage tissue, including arteries. Hydrogenation, which adds hydrogen atoms to make the polyunsaturated fat more stable at room temperature, is not healthy either.

I recommend keeping free oils to a minimum, even extra-virgin olive oil, flaxseed oil, or fish oil. Here is the main reason: Most Americans are overweight. Adding a food component that is more than twice the calories of an equivalent weight in carbohydrate or protein doesn't make a lot of sense to me. Also oils are not a very nutrient-dense food.

Water

Water is critical to human health. The majority of our bodies are water. To function properly the body requires several liters of water per day to avoid dehydration. This amount varies depending on the level of activity, temperature, humidity, and other factors. Many health experts recommend six to eight glasses of water daily as the minimum to maintain proper hydration, but the scientific backing for this recommendation is questionable. Recommendations by the Food and Nutrition Board are (including food sources) 2.7 liters of water (91 ounces, or almost three quarts) for women and 3.7 liters (125 ounces, or almost one gallon) for men daily.[13]

Periodically, even if it is for only one day, just drink water as your only fluid. See if you feel anything different that day or the next day. Sometimes the best way to really get a feel for whether something is good for you or not is to go on it completely, then off of it. Water is no exception. If you fill containers at work and at home and then put them in the refrigerator, you may be more likely to drink them than by filling up on demand.

Teas

All teas (green, white, black, Oolong) have polyphenolic antioxidant plant compounds in them called catechins, which belong to the flavonoid family. Green teas have received most of the notoriety and have been studied with positive effects on different chronic diseases, such as cardiovascular disease, cancer, and diabetes, and may even enhance fat loss. If you add a creamer or milk to the tea, however, you may be negating some of the effectiveness of these catechins.[14] Tea (black, green, or white) consumption in general may be beneficial to enhancing antioxidant protection.[15] Two to three cups of green tea has been shown to increase antioxidant capacity in a dose-dependent manner in humans.[16]

Meats (Optional)

The reason I say that meat (which includes red meats, poultry, fowl, wild game, fish, and eggs) is optional is that we can absolutely live without it, as I explained earlier.

Of course, it is your choice. As I have admitted, the healthiest cultures in the world eat small amounts of animal foods. If you do eat meat, eat free-ranged, grass-fed, antibiotic-free animals or hunted wild game. The fat in animals reflects what they are fed. Grass-fed, or grazing animals, take on the fat content of the vegetation they eat, which generally has more omega-3 fatty acids and less omega-6 fatty acids. This food consumption pattern helps create an anti-inflammatory metabolism. Obviously, the same goes for locally hunted wild game.

The need to take supplemental fish oils can be reduced dramatically if you were to eat fewer foods that concentrate omega-6 fatty acids (arachidonic acid, linoleic acid), as in meat, egg, and dairy fat especially from animals fed grain (corn, wheat, etc.) and/or soybean. We have created the great "need" for omega-3 fatty acids (EPA and DHA) from fish (or algae) because of the inflammatory, high meat-based diets rich in animal fats that usually come from factory-farmed animals fed the wrong types of fats, as well as processed foods that have the wrong types of fats.

Grocery Shopping in the *Fast Lane*

To shop healthfully is very simple and, in the right store, can be easily done in less than a half-hour with some very basic principles. While I am a big supporter of organic foods and eating seasonally and locally, I think it is incorrect to say America can't improve its health *dramatically* by shopping for non-organic whole food in the basic grocery store. To improve health, you first have to stop eating processed foods that do you no good, and even harm you, then eat quality foods that are good for you.

Principles of Grocery Shopping in the *Fast Lane*

1. Shop the outside, or "perimeter," of the grocery store where the whole, unprocessed foods are (fruit, vegetables, lean meats, etc.). Eat whole foods only (organic if possible). Buy the basics: vegetables (raw/frozen); fruit (raw/frozen); raw nuts and seeds; beans (canned/packaged); whole grains and sprouted whole grain (try non-glutinous whole grains such as brown rice, quinoa, millet, amaranth, buckwheat); water, mineral water, teas, and *real juices* (100 percent juice); animal foods (optional): eggs, fish, lean fowl, and meat (free-ranged or grass-fed if possible).

2. If you buy oils, get extra-virgin olive oil and/or cold-pressed canola oil for cooking and ground flaxseed or cold-pressed vegetable oils for salads and for cold sauces. *Keep oils to a minimum.*

3. Do not buy dairy products at all (not from a cow, goat, or sheep; not milk, cheese, yogurt, ice cream, cottage cheese, kefir, butter, etc.) for at the very least one month completely. For your whole family. *Please* don't give a child under two years of age any cow's milk products at all on a regular basis. Aside from food intolerance leading to chronic upper respiratory infections and gastrointestinal problems, of equal concern is that the early introduction of cow's milk products in children may increase the risk of type 1 diabetes, which is not reversible.[17] After the child is weaned, ideally from the mother's breast, rotate in organic almond, soy, rice, or other grain milks, fortified with calcium and vitamin D if you are concerned, *and watch* for reactions.

4. If you want a sweet, refined grain or fatty food, don't put it in your shopping cart. Go out intentionally and buy it later by itself. Only shop for whole foods and only have whole foods in your house. Build that habit and that base. Then when you choose to eat "junk," enjoy it—but not too much, and only when you are in control of your health!

Stocking Your Refrigerator and Cupboards: The Basics

Let's go to the fridge first. When you open the refrigerator, the vegetable bin should be filled with vegetables, pre-washed or fresh salad greens, spinach, chard, kale, collards—as much green, leafy vegetables as possible. Green, leafy vegetables are not only nutrient packed, but they are also 100 percent non-fattening. You are getting the most nutrients per calorie when you are eating leafy greens. Frozen vegetables are fine to have in your freezer as well.

Next, your fruit bin should always be full. I keep blackberries, blueberries, raspberries, or strawberries on one of my upper shelves, and the fruit bin is filled with whatever fruits are in season (or in the produce section), which could be apples, kiwis, nectarines, peaches, plums, oranges, grapefruit, and tangerines. I might have some bananas outside the refrigerator. For smoothies and things of that nature, it is easier to keep frozen fruit in your freezer section. Frozen is usually cheaper and you can get organic versions as well.

I keep raw nuts or seeds in the freezer. I will usually have some almonds, walnuts, pecans, and sunflower seeds. Pumpkin seeds are a very nutritous food, but for some reason don't resonate with me. Generally, I don't eat a lot of cashews and pistachios because I tend to be sensitive to them as well.

In my cupboards I always have cans of cooked beans (mostly organic) and also whole-food, organic types of soups such as minestrone, lentils, split pea, Cuban black bean, and other vegetarian things like chili. My canned products are meatless. I encourage you to do this as well. You can always add meat to them later if you must. I buy several quarts of an organic vegetarian broth to be used in soups, to stir fry, to "quick cook" my greens, or sometimes cook my pastas or grains in. (The organic vegetable broths in the quart containers have really been a lifesaver for me and revolutionized my cooking!)

It is also good to have a few quarts of marinara sauce on hand (organic is easily available). Your cooking grains can be in the cupboard or freezer, and remember that the first ingredient for any grain or flour product ideally should be "whole grain" or "sprouted grain." I usually have a loaf of sprouted, whole-grain bread in my freezer and one on the shelf in my refrigerator.

I do use, sparingly, extra-virgin olive oil (monounsaturated fat) for cooking sometimes. I have been more oil-calorie conscious lately, since really becoming aware that added oils are one of the biggest reasons for excess calories in our diet. I try to get most of my oils from nuts and seeds and avocados. If you are lean having a small amount of cold-pressed oil or spread or extra-virgin olive oil is probably fine. If you have never gone oil, nut, seed and avocado free, try it for two weeks. It is an interesting experiment. I dropped five pounds without even trying.

Have herbal teas around, especially green, black, and white teas. Mineral water can be used along with bottled or filtered water. The goal is to drink five or six glasses of water a day. If you feel you have to have some type of milky substance, there are soy, almond, and other different types of "milks," including hemp, hazelnut, oat, multigrain, and rice milks. These can all come fortified with calcium and vitamin D. Buy a variety of them and see which ones resonate with you. *When you add a new food, always ask yourself how you feel.* Even if on paper it looks good nutritionally but you don't feel well, trust that. There is always an alternative that is nutritious. Always.

If you get fish, poultry, or beef, ideally it should be wild fish and/or poultry or red meat that is grass-fed, free-ranged, and without hormones and antibiotics, or hunted game. These would round out the refrigerator.

I realize some whole-food purists, whom I respect, might look down on eating canned goods or pre-packaged, pre-washed vegetables. Ideally I'd grow my own vegetables, eat totally from my fruit trees, cook all my beans, and wash my own lettuce and greens every day, but it is not practical for me time-wise. One good thing about modern urbanization is that some businesses have done some smart things to make eating healthy in a busy world easier. By shopping and eating in this way, we can not only be healthy, but we can also help create a new, sustainable economy and jobs centered around producing whole, healthy foods that are convenient for people in the busy, modern world.

Eating out in the *Fast Lane*

Whether you eat at a fast-food restaurant or a high-end establishment, these simple guidelines can help you reduce your calories, increase your nutrient intake, and do more good than harm with meals eaten away from home.

- Avoid all creamy, cheesy sauces and dressings, and dips on any dish.
- Avoid all dairy products (cheeses, ice cream, milk, cottage cheese, sour cream, etc.). You have to ask to have dairy, especially cheese and sour cream, removed from many dishes. Presently most restaurants just add cheese and sour cream as normal fare to many foods.
- Don't order bread or chips before your meal or have them come with your meal.
- Order your salad with a dairy-free dressing on the side (vinaigrette, olive oil, etc.).
- Order plant-based appetizers if you are starved (grilled mushrooms, garlic sautéed spinach, salad rolls, lettuce cups, seaweed or cucumber salad, edamame, miso or minestrone soup, grilled vegetables, etc.).
- If you want to go completely vegetarian and there is nothing on the menu, you can just have *multiple* vegetarian appetizers, side dishes, and salads. I do this frequently.
- Ask the chef to make you a big plate full of sautéed or grilled vegetables—whatever they have available. They'll generally do it happily!
- Avoid having your food fried. Request it baked, broiled, steamed, or stir-fried. Have it light on oil, even olive oil.
- Order quick foods without added oils, salt, cheeses, mayonnaise, or sauces.
- Ask for whole-grain breads, but most restaurants don't have them.

- Replace meat with beans in fast foods when possible (on tacos, burritos, etc.). Have as many animal-free meals as possible. Leave the animal meats and products out of fast food if you can. Just ask. I do this with beans instead of meats. And of course no sour cream, cheese, mayonnaise, or creamy sauces!
- Have water instead of soda. Or have a small-sized soda with a cup of water.
- Have a pizza with the crust, tomato sauce only, and all the vegetables they want to throw on it.

The goal of eating out healthy, or doing the least amount of harm, is to keep excess calories to a minimum and eat as many unprocessed foods as possible. That is achieved by keeping creamy sauces and added oils off your basic foods; not eating lots of pre-main course snack foods; keeping high-calorie foods out of your main courses (cheeses, creamy sauces, and oils); avoiding deep fried food; avoiding alcohol; and eating as many vegetables in salads, appetizers, or in your main course, as possible.

Controlling Food Cravings

The key to controlling food cravings is to eat lots of good, whole food that gives you an even blood sugar from time-released carbohydrates and adequate protein, and has lots of fiber or natural bulk from water content. In addition, these whole foods should be *nutrient dense,* packed with lots of vitamins, minerals, antioxidants, and phytochemicals. Dr. Joel Fuhrman (*Eat to Live*, 2011) and colleagues recently showed in a study in the *Nutrition Journal* that the higher the micronutrient density of the diet, the less hunger people had while consuming fewer calories.[18] You should also keep to a minimum or eliminate foods that increase the risk of blood sugar swings (e.g., excess caffeine, simple sugars, etc.).

- Eat whole, unprocessed foods only.
- Have whole, unprocessed snacks between meals (fruit, nuts, seeds, bean spreads, whole-grain snacks).

- Eat only good, unrefined carbohydrates (beans, whole grains, fruit, starchy vegetables).
- Keep only whole foods in your house (refrigerator, cupboards).
- Go out and buy the craved food if you must. Don't have it lying around in your house.
- If you must satisfy a food craving, have it with or after a whole-food meal, not as a separate snack.
- Exercise regularly. Many times this will subdue your food cravings.
- Bring whole-food snacks to work, recreational activities, and have them in your car.
- Realize that many foods are addictive, especially ones containing simple sugars, caffeine, chocolate, dairy products, and refined grains (e.g., wheat). Avoid completely or at least take breaks from them every few days.

Conclusion

When you can't seem to digest another nutrition concept, read another label, or find the belief to trust a new fad diet, remember that a good diet is very simple. When my patients get confused, don't want to hear another diet suggestion, and their eyes are getting a bit "glazed over," I just pick out one of my favorite nutrition books of all time, *Beating The Food Giants*, and show them the front and back cover. I simply say, "Which cover of the book shows a good diet, the back or the front?" As you can see, the front cover is all refined, processed foods while the back is nothing but whole, unprocessed foods: fruits, vegetables, beans, whole grains, nuts, seeds, lean meat, fish, poultry, and eggs. It is really that simple!

Which Side is the Good Diet?

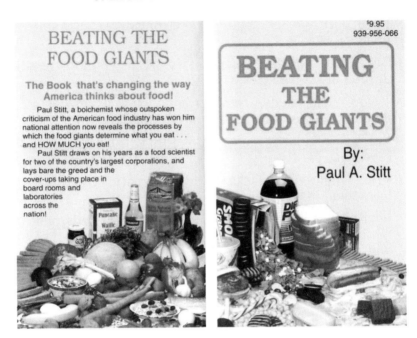

With permission from Natural Press & Barbara Stitt, *Beating the Food Giants* by Paul Stitt (1982). www.naturalpress.info/index.html

Chapter 14

THE TRIAD EXERCISE PROGRAM

Steps 4, 5, and 6 in the *9 Simple Steps to Optimal Health*

- **(Step 4) DO Aerobic Exercise** a minimum of one half-hour daily.
- **(Step 5) DO Strength Training** three to four days per week for fifteen to thirty minutes.
- **(Step 6) DO Flexibility Exercises** four to seven days per week for fifteen to sixty minutes.

Looking at any part of our human evolutionary history, there is no question that we were "born to move." All of our ancestors were moving for hours a day, working very hard, usually with the end result of feeding themselves and their kin. If we look at the modern-day "Blue Zone" populations, those enclaves of modern-day aging wonders who live and are functional into their eighties, nineties, and one hundreds, we can see that they move daily—and they move a lot! Usually hours per day doing their daily work, not minutes.

Everyone Agrees on the Importance of Exercise

Virtually no expert says that exercise isn't important for optimal health. This is one health principle you can take to the bank. The question is: How important is exercise to human health? I say critically important. You give me a regular daily exerciser as a patient, and he/she sees me less and gets well faster (usually; there are some exceptions), and generally all the therapies you try work better. So if you want to be well and stay well, stay away from doctors and hospitals, have lower medical insurance rates and bills, have more vitality, and function into your senior years then move every day! Starting *now*! Do something *daily* that gets your heart rate up (aerobics), challenges your muscles (strength training), and causes you to extend and contract ligaments, muscles, and tendons (flexibility).

"Out-of-Body" Benefits of Exercise

- Reduces individual and government healthcare costs
- Reduces health and life insurance premiums
- Increases personal and national work productivity
- Reduces prescription medication and supplement needs
- Saves money and time on medical visits and lab tests
- Gives you more energy and time to do what you enjoy

How Much Exercise Is Enough?

Thinking about how we evolved and the amount of movement done by healthy aging cultures, we need to expect movement *every day*—not three days per week, but *every day*, for a *minimum* of a half-hour per day. I say shoot for one hour daily. If you shoot for one hour and fall short a day or two, two things usually happen:

1. You don't quit being an exerciser.
2. You will continue to see results and stay motivated.

That said, remember that something is always better than nothing. If you can't hit your ideal time, do something. Fifteen minutes of walking is *always, always* better than nothing. The benefits of exercise are cumulative!

Building the "Exercise Habit"

Building the *exercise habit* is the key to incorporating this most important component of being healthy into your lifestyle. Daily structured movement has to be as important and expected as brushing your teeth, taking a shower, combing your hair, and other normal and expected activities of daily living.

When you get to the point where not exercising feels "not right," the way you'd feel if you didn't brush your teeth for the day, then you have built the *exercise habit*. When you don't go home from work until you exercise, you have built the *exercise habit*. When you don't turn on the TV before you exercise at home, or at least turn on the TV at the same time you exercise, you have built the *exercise habit*. When you are looking for ways to exercise when you are away from home on business or vacation, you have built the *exercise habit*. When you don't try to make an excuse for not exercising, you have built the *exercise habit*. If you say, "Some exercise is better than no exercise" when you can't do your regular exercise routine, and you do something else involving movement, you have developed the *exercise habit*.

It's about Time and Consistency
More than Intensity and Technique

If you are new to the exercise game, it is going to take three to nine months before you build the *exercise habit* and it becomes "part of you." The first step is to create the space (time) to exercise. Fifteen to thirty minutes is acceptable to start. The second step is to shoot for *daily* exercise. It doesn't matter at first what type of exercise, as long as it is some type of aerobic, big muscle-moving exercise and *is safe*. Build the consistency. Success with exercise is more about consistency and time than it is about technique and intensity.

If you build in the time to exercise as part of your normal day and are consistent with your exercise program, you will see results and will naturally start to pick up the intensity and duration of the exercise after a few weeks. But "pain is no gain." Some hard-core exercisers will disagree with me on this. For the average person it is far more important to have lots of victories to keep your exercise program alive than to push through pain and injure yourself or be so sore you quit. Nagging injuries, persistent soreness, and pain are "killers" to building the *exercise habit*. Down the road, after exercising three months to a year, if you really want to push yourself, give it a try. You are less likely to quit when you have built the exercise habit.

Making Exercise Efficient

Let's face it: Most of us are very busy. The most common excuse I get in the clinic is "I can't exercise because I am too busy (and/or too tired)." If you knew you were going to get results fast, you might not give that excuse so easily. I can tell you how to be efficient with your time and get results fast. How can I say this? Because I live it! I am very efficient with my exercise from strength training to aerobics and my flexibility work. I block out anywhere from one half-hour to two hours per day for exercise. Remember the **TRIAD Exercise** concept. You want to have a good cardiovascular system, be strong, and be flexible—and you want to do the exercises fast, efficiently, and *safely*.

When you have that exerciser's mentality—when that exercise habit is part of you—you will see the opportunities within your daily life to exercise efficiently and safely. You just find a way as you go through your busy day. If you get injured you find a way to exercise around it.

How to Increase "Non-Exercise" Exercise

More traditional cultures get their exercise from "non-exercise" exercise. Just the work they have to do to feed themselves, their daily jobs, and taking care of their dwellings provide some vigorous physical activity. The modern-day American who sits all day at work, comes home and eats, and then sits and watches TV an average of five hours per day should do as much "non-exercise" exercise as possible *and* do planned exercise daily to get close to what healthy aging cultures do automatically.[1]

Since time is precious to all of us, it is very important that we make exercise time-efficient and as fun as possible. One way is to do as much "non-exercise" exercise as possible. Let's look at a few examples:

> Get up off the couch and change the TV channel instead of using the remote control.

> Get up for five to ten minutes for each hour of sitting. Use breaks to walk or stretch.

> If you watch television, *do aerobic exercise in front of your favorite television show* daily. This could change America's health dramatically! Virtually overnight!

> Do isometrics periodically while sitting (contracting and relaxing of muscles) or, better yet, pick up some dumb bells while sitting (and use them!). If you are older and all you have is canned products around, use the cans as dumb bells.

> Restrict sitting to activities that require it, such as eating, learning, writing, keyboarding, and essential driving.

> Sit on a ball while at your home or at work instead of a traditional chair.

> Walk briskly while doing chores, shopping, or errands.

> Do your own gardening or mow your own lawn.

> Take the stairs versus the elevator or escalator.

> Walk in an airport instead of using the moving walkway.

> Park in the parking lot in a *far away* spot. Don't drive around to get the closest spot.

➢ Walk to a local restaurant around your work place at lunch.

➢ Ride your bicycle or walk to work.

➢ Walk to public transit and use it versus hopping into your car.

➢ Any time you use a device (car, escalator, stairs, etc.) to take the "walk" out of walking, just walk—within reason. We are talking about a few extra minutes, not hours, because you choose to walk.

These activities add up. The benefits of movement are cumulative. I have heard some very successful weight-loss specialists talk about how important it is to get obese people to add this "non-exercise" exercise to a structured exercise program. One physician who was a weight-loss specialist also did hospital work. He committed himself to using the stairs during his hospital rounds versus the elevator and was amazed at how much exercise he got while seeing patients in his very busy medical practice.

Just think: These basic examples only cover the simple things we can do as a part of our daily routines. They don't even begin to account for all the exercise opportunities just waiting to be incorporated into our "fun" time!

Exercising when Traveling for Business or Pleasure

When staying at a hotel, always ask if there is a fitness room. Hopefully it is free, but even if you have to pay to use it, it is worth it! Trips can be stressful enough (whether for business or pleasure), so it's critical to have a space to exercise, take a little edge off, and do something good for your body. Just because the setup is different or less optimal than your home or personal gym, be creative. You can *always* adapt and get in a workout. Remember: *Something is always better than nothing!* By not skipping a day when traveling, even if you do less than you normally do, you are more likely to stay with your overall program and ultimately be successful in your fitness goals.

If the hotel does not have an exercise room, look for a space in your room to stretch and do push-ups, chair-dips, etc. I find a space in my hotel room to do a little yoga or even practice some dance steps, listening to a salsa CD or do my *Rodney Yee's A.M. Yoga for Your Week* DVD (Gaiam Americas Inc, 2008) from my computer for fifteen minutes. It is not my perfect workout, but it is much better than nothing. Bring one or two of your favorite exercise DVDs and plug them into your laptop if you brought one. Also, ask the concierge or front-desk staff if there is a safe place to walk around the hotel.

On a cruise or at an all-inclusive resort, check out the gym and see if there are any classes you might like to sign up for (yoga, aerobics, dance, etc.) or go work out.

If there is something physically active you like to do (dancing, swimming, snorkeling, boogie boarding, hiking, aerobics, yoga, etc.), find it where you are traveling! It's easy in this modern world: Just Google the city name and the activity. I'm a dancer, so I always check out salsa and lindy hop dance venues near where I am going on vacation or business.

If your vacation is outdoors and near nature, hiking and swimming are enjoyable and productive ways to exercise.

Even if you can't keep up your normal routine when away, **do something!** Remember that **exercise is cumulative**. You won't lose that much from your regular fitness routine if you do something while away from home.

The TRIAD Exercise Program

I recommend what I call the **TRIAD Exercise Program**, which is simple, *time-efficient*, and *safe*. These are steps 4, 5, and 6 of the *9 Simple Steps to Optimal Health*:

TRIAD Exercise *Phase I* (Step 4): Efficient Aerobics

DO a minimum of one half-hour **DAILY** with a goal of one hour daily of aerobic exercise.

Aerobic exercise is simply moving your big muscles (legs, arms, etc.) and getting your heart rate up to where you can still talk, but you are breathing and hopefully breaking a sweat. If you haven't been exercising in a while and/or are overweight or have cardiac issues, you should see your doctor first.

> ➤ Incorporate your exercise into as much of your normal daily duties as possible. Think about it: How much of your normal daily activity can you make into movement?

> ➤ Walk with a family member or your entire family. I can't think of anything more important than exercising and spending quality time with your family; it is a "win-win."

> ➤ Do recreational things outside your home that can include your family member(s) or spouse and that also include *aerobic* movement: hiking, walking the dog, pushing a stroller, speed walking with a child in a backpack, ballroom dancing, etc. *Move with those you love.*

> ➤ If you are stuck at home because of family duties, weather, or safety, exercise in front of the TV. Set an example for your children and your spouse. *Make it a priority!* Don't turn on the TV until you get on your favorite piece of exercise equipment.

> ➤ Do a DVD of some kind of aerobic/dance program at home before the kids get up or after they go to bed.

> ➤ Make sure you get up and move at least every hour if you have a sit-down job.

> ➤ You can also break up the activity in one session (ten minutes stair-stepper, ten minutes treadmill, ten minutes elliptical rider). The combination isn't important; keeping

yourself from getting bored and moving for at least thirty minutes is important!

➤ Don't be stuck on one movement activity for aerobics. Exercise is cumulative. You could exercise for fifteen minutes on the stair-stepper at your business gym and then walk with your family/spouse for a half-hour when you get home. Or maybe go to a martial arts class in the evening or dance for an hour (keep a vision in the back of your mind of a total goal of one hour per day).

➤ Rotate aerobic exercises so you don't get bored. For example, play tennis two days per week, walk two days, take an aerobics class two days, and hike one day. Do something every day!

➤ Walk wherever you can walk during your normal working day. (Skip escalators, elevators, short car rides, parking close, etc.)

➤ If you are a bit crazy like me, keep your running shoes and exercise shorts in the trunk of your car. Change in the gym parking lot or near a park (discreetly, of course!), and go run or walk.

➤ Be creative. Ask yourself throughout your day where you can be more active. You will see opportunities. Take them.

➤ Then say to yourself, "Wow! I am improving my health, saving money, reducing my risk of serious disease, feeling better, looking better, becoming the director of my health, and investing in the best Fortune 500 company ever: ME!"

TRIAD Exercise *Phase II* (Step 5): Efficient Strength Training

DO safe and efficient **strength training** fifteen to thirty minutes three to four days per week.

First and foremost, you don't have to spend hours in the gym to get a really cut body and be strong. People make it way too difficult and complicated. I see it every time I go to the gym. With a focused, fifteen-minute circuit training program three to four days per week, you can have a great physique and be strong. It may sound egotistical, but I know it because I do it, and I get compliments on my fifty-plus-year-old body frequently.

To do it you have to be consistent and efficient. You don't have to kill yourself, but you need to work hard to get results fast. You also have to eat right and get lean if you want your physique to show definition. You don't need to be downing protein-rich sports drinks, or eating tons of meat and eggs daily or immediately after exercising. Just eat the whole food. If you choose to have animal foods, which are not necessary for muscles or for good health, then eat lean meat, poultry (grass-fed, free-ranged, hormone- and antibiotic-free), and fish in the context of your three daily meals surrounded by lots of unrefined plant foods. You meat-eating and dairy-supplementing gym rats have been duped into thinking you have to consume lots of protein and animal foods to be strong and athletic. Also I am not aware of any study that shows being big increases longevity.

This reminds me of an acquaintance I'd see working out in the gym. He was a big, thick, muscular guy who lifted a fair amount of weight. He was telling me about his weight issues and medical problems with diabetes, hypertension, and kidney issues. He was a classic "dairy-aholic" and was stunned when I told him to eliminate the dairy, cut back on the meat, and eat more vegetables, and that he'd still be fine in the gym. I also told him he'd drop some weight and probably improve his diabetes and kidney function. He was fearful of not being strong and muscular if he cut back on those foods (meat and dairy, to which he was addicted).

Americans have been brainwashed by the propaganda that you have to consume meat, poultry, fish, and dairy products to be healthy and strong. It's complete B.S.! This belief has hurt—and will continue to hurt—a lot of people who think this.

Circuit Training for Strength

The average modern person is very busy. He or she doesn't have hours and hours to train in the gym, is not an elite athlete training for some type of competition, and is not a movie star trying to tweak a particular area of his or her body. That said, building lean body mass is not only healthy for our metabolism (blood sugar control and immune function), but also helps us function in our daily lives, especially as we get older. I am a *big fan* of circuit training. It is fast; there are no weights to put away; it is **safe**; you don't need a partner or coach; it works different muscle groups in their full range of motion; it works the body symmetrically; it is easy for anyone to use after maybe one or two sessions of instruction; and it has some cardiovascular benefit (not a lot) if you keep moving.

You can get a very efficient workout in fifteen to thirty minutes. I included fifteen minutes because that is what it takes me: fifteen minutes at a consistent pace to do six different upper-body exercises and six lower-body exercises.

Just do circuit training in the above-mentioned fashion for two months (along with a whole-food, plant-strong diet). If you want to speed up the process, do the circuit training every other day for a month. If you want to spend twenty-five to thirty minutes doing circuit training, do just ten to twelve different upper-body exercises and ten to twelve different lower-body exercises. The key is moving steadily between stations; alternate arm and leg exercises so you don't fatigue a group of muscles. Do as many different exercises as the machines allow before repeating an exercise so you work as many different muscle groups and go through as many different ranges of motion as possible. Keep the number of sets of exercises even between the upper and lower body to help keep some balance between the strength and bulk in our lower bodies compared to our upper bodies. Do ten to fifteen repetitions with each exercise. When you can do fifteen or more repetitions easily, try increasing the weight, number of plates, or resistance on the machines. Likewise, if ten repetitions are too strenuous, decrease the weight.

This is not the only way to strength train by any means, but it works for busy people and gets results *fast* and *safely*. That is the focus of this book. My goal is to give you fast, efficient, and safe ways to get to a very high state of health with minimal expense and time in your busy, modern lifestyle. The great thing about weight training is that you get results. It is black and white. If you lose weight at the same time, you will become doubly excited about seeing the fat go away and the curves come out of *nowhere!*

I recommend warming up with your aerobic exercises prior to your circuit training to allow the muscles to be warm and have some blood flow going through them before challenging them. Then do anywhere from ten to thirty minutes of stretching after your circuit training. After doing this routine several months, you may adapt your warm-up and stretching any way you feel comfortable. Just listen to your body! I repeat: **listen to your body!** It will tell you when you have to rest, ease up, or push yourself a bit more.

I am not against free weights. Circuit training with machines is just fast and efficient and can get you results quickly. (For the record, I do curls and bench press with free weights in my routine, have a pull-up bar, and bar dip setup at home.) You can do similar workouts with free weights. It may take a bit more time setting up the weights.

As I mentioned, for fast results I would do the circuit training every other day for a month or two. For older individuals, the muscle recovery may not be as quick, and every other day may create some extra soreness. Just be cautious of this. If you're too sore, don't push yourself as hard and still go every other day, or put two days in between your circuit training regularly or periodically, depending on your soreness. Just be consistent.

Getting "Gorilla Buff" Fast

Why do I use the term "Gorilla Buff?" Because gorillas don't eat other animals to get their protein and they are big and muscular. It is true that some species of gorillas, especially lowland gorillas, eat a fair amount of ants and termites (maybe up to 3 percent of their diet) and get protein and certain trace minerals from these insects, but the bulk of their protein comes from massive quantities of leafy plant foods, stems, bark, and fruit when available. Mountain gorillas tend to have a more limited diet and eat fewer termites, ants and fruit, and more leafy foliage and other vegetation.[2] Gorillas may also eat certain plant foods to prevent infections from parasites and other conditions.[3]

Interestingly, this conclusion was made by world-renowned physician-researcher and developer of the Glycemic Index Dr. David Jenkins and colleagues after studying the diets of western lowland gorillas: "...The macronutrient profile of this diet would be as follows: 2.5% energy as fat, 24.3% protein, 15.8% available carbohydrate, with potentially 57.3% of metabolizable energy from short-chain fatty acids (SCFA) derived from colonic fermentation of fiber. Gorillas would therefore obtain considerable energy through fiber fermentation. We suggest that humans also evolved consuming similar high foliage, high fiber diets, which were low in fat and dietary cholesterol."[4]

If a gorilla can build massive muscles from eating almost all plant foods, so can you—especially if you add beans, nuts, seeds, and whole grains to your large vegetable and fruit intake. If you want to get "Gorilla Buff" fast, it isn't all in the strength training you do. It is in the diet and, to a lesser extent, the aerobic exercise you do. Building muscle under a layer of fat is still building muscle, but it isn't getting the shape or the look you want. If you are overweight, you want to eat whole foods, although you might stay away from or reduce consumption of even whole-grain breads for a while since they are more calorie dense (see Chapter 13, Reducing Caloric Density) than eating the basic cooked grains until you lean out. Get rid of any added oils and sugar. Excess calories from any source will get turned to fat.

You want to lose the weight while you build muscle underneath. If overweight, do a daily aerobic program for thirty to sixty minutes, along with your every-other-day, fifteen- to thirty-minute circuit training program (six to ten upper-body exercises and six to ten lower-body exercises); and a ten- to fifteen-minute (or more) flexibility program daily for one or two months. If you want to spend more time in the gym, just increase the time of the aerobics, number of exercises for your circuit training, and duration of stretching.

You should make your gym experience one continuous exercise. Don't stop, chitchat, or rest. Just keep moving! You will see rapid results. *Don't* overeat protein or fat calories! This is not necessary and can be harmful!

Keep a picture of a four-hundred-pound muscular gorilla in your mind eating tons of greens and fruit, plus a few termites or ants, if you don't believe you can be muscular eating lots of plant foods. In fact, the January 2008 issue of *National Geographic* (pp. 88–105) featured an article on these magnificent creatures. One photo shows a large male sitting in a pond "sucking down" some type of green plant, stem first (p. 99)!

So the next time someone asks you where do you get your protein for muscles by eating only plant foods, ask them where do you think a gorilla gets its muscles (and the elephant, hippo, giraffe, and, yes, the cow)? Tell them the answer is in the January 2008 issue of *National Geographic* on page 99!

Strength Training for the Elderly—a Must!

We are aging, and aging fast, in the United States (and the world). We have to stay functional. Exercise in our seniors is critical for a viable economy and healthcare system. Strength training is very important in this group to maintain function and independence and keep healthcare costs reasonable.

In my older patients, I am even more adamant about strength training. They think I am a bit crazy, but they appreciate it when they get my "sense of urgency" for them to do some form of strength training so they can remain as **independent** as possible for as long as they can. The number one concern of older people, from my experience, is the worry and desire to remain **independent**.

I think my older patients also appreciate that I don't expect them to be falling apart. I expect them to be slowing the aging process. I expect them to really improve their strength and physical well-being. Most of them haven't been told they can improve their physical condition. We need to *expect* our elderly to be strong, fit, and functional until the day they die. Aging isn't about being "put out to pasture." It is about staying active, vibrant, strong, and contributing to their communities.

We tend to focus most on aerobic exercise, which is appropriate. But the value of strength training as we grow older to help maintain body metabolism, our *independence,* strength, and overall bodily functions is critical. It may be the most important exercise component of all. When muscle mass is lost with aging due to lack of exercise (hormones and nutrition), bad things happen. In addition, as we get older, flexibility becomes more and more important. Flexibility is essential to help prevent us from falling, straining things, creating injuries, and other problems that can make us more sedentary. Let's talk about keeping your muscles as we age.

One of my favorite examples of this that speaks a thousand words is a CNN report entitled, "Secret of Long Life In Okinawa." Play this three-minute You Tube video clip.[5] You will see a ninety-year-old female Okinawan elder climbing a big citrus tree and filling up a large basket of fruit. She has been working on this farm for seventy years, and she works eight hours per day picking fruit. It also shows Okinawan elders exercising and dancing together, running races, and of course eating whole unprocessed food, a lot of which are plant foods.

Like all healthy aging cultures with remarkable longevity, physical activity resembling a type of natural cross-training is part of their normal day. Many of us in the West have to put these activity habits by intention into our busy lives. This ninety-year-old tree-climbing wonder is one of my favorite examples of healthy aging and the "use it or lose it" axiom!

Now take another three minutes and watch a sequel to this clip entitled "Western Diet: A Killer in Okinawa."[6] This CNN report shows that the long-living elders in Okinawa who live the traditional healthy lifestyle may be "dying out" because the next two generations of Okinawans are eating the fast food, highly processed Western diet filled with little physical activity. They have the highest rates of obesity and heart disease anywhere in Japan. These three-minute video clips show the causes and the answers to our healthcare crisis and real healthcare reform in the United States and world.

It's not genetics or the need for a new medical discovery and billions of dollars in research. It's lifestyle: diet, exercise, and how we relate to each other in community. And we already have the knowledge and examples. We just have to do it. *It is that simple!* It is not up to the politicians. Every bit of this is in your hands right now! That's right. *I am calling each one of you out right now!* You know how to create individual healthcare reform right now. If we all do it then the healthcare crisis vanishes and along with it, the economic woes related to worker's health, healthcare expense, productivity, and our national economy.

What Does *"Sar-co-PEE-nee-ah"* Have to Do with Healthy Aging?

There is a medical condition called sarcopenia. It means loss of skeletal muscle mass and a reduction in the metabolic quality of muscle in the elderly.[7]

Sarcopenia begins around the age of forty-five, when muscle mass begins to decline at a rate of about 1 percent a year.[8] The amount of muscle mass lost in the elderly is directly related to the loss of strength, which is the main cause of increased disability in the elderly. Muscle strength is a critical component for walking and balance. The high prevalence of falls in the elderly is directly related to the reduction in lower-body strength.[9]

The following excerpt taken from an interview I did with Dr. Chad M. Kerksick, director of the Applied Biochemistry and Molecular Physiology Laboratory, Department of Health and Exercise Science at the University of Oklahoma, punctuates the seriousness of sarcopenia as a public health problem.

"...Over time my research interests have shifted from the enhancement of sport performance to maintaining skeletal muscle mass with age in an attempt to improve the quality and duration of life. I found it appalling that approximately 20% of Americans ≥ 60 years of age are classified as functionally disabled as a result of skeletal muscle loss, and direct health care costs associated with muscle loss that occurs with aging costs the United States government $18.5 billion in 2000."[10]

One esteemed researcher who has championed strength training in the elderly for several decades is Dr. William Evans, the director of the Nutrition, Metabolism, and Exercise Laboratory in the Donald Reynolds Department of Geriatrics at the University of Arkansas for Medical Sciences. Very clearly he has shown that sarcopenia can be slowed and reversed with weight/strength training in the elderly. Yes, even those in their nineties can build muscle![11]

Why is this important? You need strong muscles for daily physical activity and *remaining independent*—the ability to climb stairs, do chores, dance, take walks, take care of your garden, enjoy a day out sight-seeing, get in and out of your car, grocery shop, clean your house, and many other activities of daily living. An added bonus from resistance training is that building lean body mass helps with blood sugar and weight control. Lean muscle burns more energy than fat![12]

The rates of population growth for those over the ages of sixty to sixty-five around the world are greater than the rate of growth of the general population.[13] So we better get our rapidly expanding aging population as functional and independent for as long as possible, because there is no healthcare system in the world that can take care of all the chronic diseases that will occur if the world keeps going in the direction it is going.

As much as I am a believer in aerobic exercise, it will not necessarily prevent sarcopenia from happening. If natural strength building is not part of your normal daily activities, as it is in many traditional aging societies, you need to program it in. Strength training is a critical part of wellness, anti-aging, possibly cancer prevention, and protecting the viability of our healthcare system.

Home "Pearls of Wisdom"
for the Elderly to Stay Strong

The elderly can do everything I have recommended for anyone strength training if they go to a gym or have an in-home gym, but here are a few suggestions for home application when you don't have a gym or are housebound:

> ➤ Get up and down from your chair at least five to twenty times each hour. You don't have to walk anywhere. Just get up and sit down. You can do "sets" of five to twenty at the end of each TV show or each half-hour. This helps thigh strength and arm strength.

> ➤ Do chair bar-dips—any amount, every hour. You don't have to leave the chair. Just try to push yourself up using the arm rests (careful the arm rests don't break!).

> ➤ If you have dumb bells, keep them next to where you sit. Do sets in all the directions that you can move your arms with every hour of sitting. Use cans of beans or soup if you don't have dumb bells.

> ➤ Do straight leg raises or knee extensions from your chair. Hold your legs out for five to twenty seconds every hour. Put small weights on your ankles for more resistance.

> ➤ Do calf raises or quarter-squats holding onto the door frame or a chair, or do "sink squats" by holding onto the sink and squatting gently with no joint pain (never more than ninety degrees). Put a non-rolling chair underneath your butt to prevent falling. (Safety first! Prevent falls!)

> ➤ Do angled push-ups against the wall or a countertop.

Here is one way to apply the **TRIAD Exercise Program** to the elderly when allocating their time to exercise: one-third aerobic, one-third strength training, and one-third flexibility. Just give equal time to each discipline. But most importantly keep moving your body, all parts of it! In the elderly, it is more important to live by the popular phrase "use it or lose it!"

TRIAD Exercise *Phase III* (Step 6): Efficient Flexibility Training

DO SOME type of **flexibility exercises** four to seven days per week for fifteen to sixty minutes. In fact, any way you look at it, flexibility needs to be incorporated into your **TRIAD Exercise Program** for some or all of the following reasons:

- To keep you limber so you can do the normal activities of daily living with ease.
- To prevent repetitive-use injuries to muscles, tendons, and joints that you use frequently for work, daily function, or recreation.
- To prevent back pain and help preserve what spinal disk integrity is left with the pumping of fluid in and out of the disk area.
- To prevent shoulder and neck pain and headaches from the chronic tension caused by the sedentary lifestyle of the aging Westerner.
- To de-stress you and provide a sense of relaxation and peace.
- To allow you to keep doing the other two phases of the **TRIAD Exercise Program** (aerobics and strength training).

Here are some "flexibility pearls" for this important third phase of the **TRIAD Exercise Program** or sixth *Step to Optimal Health.*

➤ Do some light aerobics or your aerobic workout before you stretch, if possible. It generally feels better to stretch with warm muscles.

➤ Always ease into your flexibility exercises: stretching, yoga, or Pilates training.

➤ Do a short, fifteen- to twenty-minute yoga, Pilates, tai chi, or qi gong DVD if you don't have the time for an hour or hour-and-a-half class (www.gaiam.com is an excellent re-source for such DVDs). Clear a space in your house for this. Get a yoga mat and cloth belt to assist you in stretching.

➤ Do safe, secure, light stretching in the shower when the hot water is running on the areas of stretch.

➤ Stretch in a pool or a hot tub.

➤ When sitting for long periods of time while traveling, stand up and stretch at your seat or go to the back of the plane. If driving, pull over at a rest stop and get out of the car to stretch.

➤ Use walls anywhere to do flexion and extension of your lower back. Just stand arm's length from a wall (palms on the wall), feet shoulder-width apart, and move your pelvis toward the wall. Then move your pelvis away while flexing forward with palms still flat on the wall. Repeat this five to twenty times.

➤ Stretch on the floor while watching TV.

➤ If you have no idea how to stretch, get the book *Stretching* by Bob and Jean Anderson (2010). It's a classic. (The thirtieth anniversary edition just came out.)

➤ Remember that any stretching is better than no stretch-ing.

➤ If you get muscle cramps, try supplementing with calcium and magnesium in a one-to-one ratio at 500 mg each or at a dose that doesn't give you loose stools from the ex-tra magnesium (especially if you just got off dairy prod-ucts). Hold your caffeinated beverages (coffees, teas, en-ergy drinks, soft drinks, etc.). They can aggravate muscle cramps. If it is hot and you sweat a lot, you may also add salt to your food.

➤ Doing any exercise or recreation that moves a wide vari-ety of muscles and limbs in different ways is very help-ful for flexibility and can be a natural way of stretching (dancing, martial arts, basketball, etc).

Simple Exercises to Keep Backs Pain Free

By doing simple, gentle, pain-free flexion-extension exercises, simple trunk rotation, and hamstring exercises consistently, many lower back problems can be prevented. (NOTE: *No matter what any health professional tells you (me included), if it hurts, DO NOT DO IT! Go "up to" and around back pain, but do not push through it!*) Here are some simple back exercises you can do.

➢ Try to do some form of flexion-extension exercises every day, even if it is just for a few minutes. If you are standing, "flexion" is bending forward from the waist, and "extension" is tilting backward from the waist (try not to curve your back but bend at the waist).

➢ Do some hamstring stretches (back of your thighs between your butt and knees) every day.

➢ Do some type of large muscle movement every day—a non-traumatic aerobic exercise. Backs love big muscle movement. Do an activity that *doesn't hurt* your back, but do something.

➢ "Wake your back up" in the morning before getting out of bed, especially if you have a sore back. (1) Pull your knees up with feet flat on the bed and rock your knees (together) gently from side to side. Gently, complete a greater rotation with each rocking motion. (2) Lift your pelvis up to the ceiling, as if you had a string tied to your navel and you were a puppet with someone gently pulling the string from above. Then let it come down and repeat five to ten times. (3) Pull each knee toward your chest. (4) Then pull both knees to your chest. Do these simple stretches five to ten times each. (5) Roll to your side and slide off the bed to either a standing position or to your knees. (6) If on all "fours," do the "angry cat" stretch: Arch your back like an angry cat, then let it go down like a sway back in an old horse with your face looking up. Then gently tilt your pelvis between those two movements five to ten times.

➢ Have a towel or belt (cloth belt/strap is best) to loop around the arch of your foot so you can keep your back straight if you are lying on the ground while flexing your straight leg up and forward at the waist to do a hamstring stretch. If sitting on the ground with straightened legs, you can loop the towel or belt over your arches as extensions of your arms and bend forward from the waist. Don't curve your back. These stretch your hamstrings and lower back.

➢ Standing with your feet at least shoulder-width apart, begin to move your hips in a circular motion to the right for five to ten rotations and then to the left. Keep your feet planted in the same place throughout.

➢ Don't sit for more than a half-hour without getting up if possible (desk, chair, car, plane, etc.).

➢ Sit on a large, air-filled medicine ball at your home or work instead of a chair (I have to thank Dr. Stella Volpe, professor and chair, Drexel University, Department of Nutrition for this suggestion. The final stages of this book were written sitting for hours on such a medicine ball in my home office).

➢ If you jog, have good shoes. Put some type of cushion and/ or arch support in your shoe to see if it helps with your legs and back. Jog on softer surfaces such as grass or dirt, or do other exercises like a stair master, stepper, elliptical rider, etc., that are less traumatic on your back.

➢ Do wall flexion and extension exercises, or what I call "Wall Yoga" while standing up. Spread your feet shoulder-width apart, with palms flat against the wall directly in front of you at shoulder level. Let your pelvis sink toward the wall with legs straight and your head tilted gently back, only if comfortable (modified Upward Dog). Hold for five to ten seconds, then walk your hands down the wall so your butt sticks out, you are flexed forward at the hips with your legs straight, and your arms are stretched at your head level or above (modified Downward Dog). You will feel a stretch in your low back, hamstrings, and shoulders. Hold for five to ten seconds, and repeat. Do this complete motion five to ten times. It can be done anywhere there is a wall, from the inside of an airplane to the side of your car. This is a great way to keep your lower back loose. If you sit all day, do *wall yoga* every half-hour or hour throughout the day, with five to twenty pumping actions alternating between flexion and extension. Just three to five minutes one to three times daily can make a world of difference in your back health. Remember: if it hurts your back don't do it—*pain is no gain with backs!*

➤ Shoulder Walk: Hold onto a door jamb or put your palm flat on the wall, with fingers pointed in the same direction as the arm that you are using (right arm, fingers pointing to your right; left arm, fingers pointing to the left) at shoulder level with arms extended. Slowly turn your torso away from the direction of your arm so you stretch the front part of your shoulder socket. Keep turning gently your total torso away from the arm that is placed palm-flat against the wall until you feel a nice stretch. Then switch arms and turn the other way, stretching the other shoulder.

➤ *Gently,* with legs straight (or one straight and one slightly bent), bend forward *from the waist,* and try to touch your toes or come close. Do not strain or curl your back. Then come up with hands on hips and arch backward with feet planted. Tilt the pelvis forward and head backward with an arch in your back that is a comfortable stretch (*no pain*). Hold five to ten times, and repeat gently.

➤ Do something at least daily, or preferably several times per day, for your back. Daily exercises and stretches, even for five minutes a day, can keep a "bad back" a non-issue.

➤ Lay down for five to ten minutes on the floor with your legs from the back of your knees to your heels resting on a chair (or cushions) while you lay with back flat on the ground and your knees and hips at ninety degrees. Just rest. This is one of the simplest and most effective back relieving techniques. You don't have to do anything. Just lay in that position.

> Do *no-pain* tai chi, yoga, or Pilates four to seven days per week.

> Again, don't ever push your back! If it hurts, don't do it! Work up to the pain and around it, but not through it!

Common Back Pain: Things You Can Do Now!

> Exercise *pain free,* as above.

> Eat off the BED list for two to four weeks or, if you do no other dietary change, at least get off **all** milk products (cheese, ice cream, milk, yogurt, sour cream, kefir) for one month. (see Appendix A). Yes! Food intolerance can cause back (and joint) pain. Especially dairy and wheat.

> Eliminate for two to four weeks all caffeine beverages (including caffeine-containing medications).

> Some nutrients that may help your back: vitamin D 2,000–6,000 IU/day (get a blood level; optimal 40–70 ng/ml); calcium 500–1,000 mg/d; magnesium 500–1,000 mg/d (watch for loose stools at high dose; elderly must have good kidney function); B complex 50–100 mg/d; glucosamine HCL 1,000–3,000 mg/d; fish oil 3,000–5,000 mg/d EPA/DHA or vegan DHA 400-1000 mg (algal oil); ginger 1–2 gm/d; curcumin 500–1,000 mg/d.

TV and Exercise: America's Way to Healthcare Reform?

Americans watch a lot of TV, as reported by The Nielsen Company in their *Three Screen Report* in 2009.

"The typical American continues to increase his/her media time, watching each week almost 35 hours of TV, 2 hours of time-shifted TV, 22 minutes of online video and 4 minutes of mobile video, while also spending 4 hours on the Internet." From the fourth quarter in 2009 to the first quarter in 2010, the average hours:minutes watched per month increased from 153:47 to 158:25.[14]

That's five hours per day of television and more than 150 hours per month! If Americans exercised daily for one-tenth (thirty minutes) or one-fifth (one hour) of the time they were watching television per day on some type of aerobic machine—*Game Over!*—the most dramatic public health improvement ever accomplished in the United States would occur. This wouldn't cost anybody a dime except the initial investment in some kind of exercise machine. (If the government could prove you exercised during your television watching at least a half-hour, the equipment should be tax deductible or there should be some type of rebate! I mean this sincerely.) No extra time would be taken out from your precious day. Millions if not billions of dollars in healthcare costs could be saved from this simple campaign. Just think—if we added a whole-food diet to this national campaign of exercising while watching television! Voila! Healthcare reform is a moot point!

So don't ever tell me you watch television but don't have time to exercise—that is **not** an excuse! If you have a favorite television show and you watch television daily, you should purchase something like a stair-stepper, rebounder, treadmill, exercycle, or elliptical rider (whatever) and put it in front of the TV (not garage or spare bedroom!). When you first turn on the television for your favorite show, get on whatever piece of equipment you have and stay on it for the duration of that show minimally. Even if you can't afford to purchase some type of exercise equipment, if you just stand up and then sit down from your couch or chair continuously for a half-hour for just one show, or stepped in place, that would dramatically change the health of this country. **It is that simple!**

Recently, I had a seventy-year-old patient who was so proud that she had walked on the treadmill during a half-hour of the *Oprah* show five days per week (as I had been harping on for months!). I said, "Oprah's show is an hour. Why only thirty minutes?!" Then I asked, "What show are you going to watch on the weekends to exercise every day?" She and I laughed, but I was dead serious. Use it or lose it. Especially in the elderly, exercise *every* day! Shoot for an hour!

You may have a greater chance of building the exercise habit if you use your favorite TV show as the "cue" for doing your daily exercise. This is part of being efficient and making your health a fun part-time job.

TRIAD Exercise Program: Conclusions

I hope I have made it abundantly clear how critically important exercise is to your overall health, yet how simple it is to incorporate it into different parts of your daily living. The real key is to build the *exercise habit*. Take three to nine months to build this important wellness pillar. Once it is part of you, and you incorporate it daily into your life in fun, creative ways, it is not work anymore and you are truly living the principle "make your health a fun part-time job." You will be reaping the benefits for a lifetime.

Remember, do something daily, but don't hurt yourself. Incorporate the **TRIAD Exercise Program's** three phases of aerobics, strength, and flexibility into your daily routine. Congratulate yourself for adding this exercise program to your excellent health insurance program (**TRIAD Wellness Program**). The great thing about exercise is this: if you just do it—if you just put in the time—you are guaranteed results. *Guaranteed!* You don't have to be a rocket scientist or an elite athlete; you just have to do it. You always get results. And when you add the dietary steps previously mentioned, the results come faster and are longer lasting.

Chapter 15

THE TRIAD MIND-BODY PROGRAM

Steps 7, 8, and 9 in the *9 Simple Steps to Optimal Health*

- **(Step 7) BE thankful** for five minutes morning and evening.
- **(Step 8) SIT quietly** for fifteen to sixty minutes daily.
- **(Step 9) IMAGINE your ideal health and life** daily five to fifteen minutes. Think about what you want, not about what you don't want. Write it down. Picture it!

In this book, we have talked about things that are very biochemical (**TRIAD Diet Program**) and biomechanical (**TRIAD Exercise Program**) and how they can affect your health. Now we are going to enter the last and most powerful phase of wellness, the **TRIAD Mind-Body Program.**

While most people, deep down, recognize that the mind is the most powerful part of us, generally it is the least talked about because it is hard to quantify your improvement and progress. It's not like pounds coming off from healthy dieting. Nor is it as evident as working with weights and seeing that muscle definition develop or doing aerobics and seeing improvement in miles on the treadmill or seeing your body become more flexible. Your improvement with mind-body training can be that you just feel better and are more relaxed and that life is flowing—it's kind of hard to measure.

In this discussion of the third and final leg of the **TRIAD Wellness Program**, we start with things that can affect the mind biochemically, then move into the more subtle but most powerful aspects of health, healing, and living a happy life. After all, the goal of all this is to live a happy, purposeful life—one of service and self-fulfillment.

Helping the Mind's Biochemistry

- Control blood sugar – Eat low-glycemic, whole, unprocessed foods (glycemic index ≤ 55, glycemicindex.com).
- Minimize stimulants and medications – Caffeine, smoking, and recreational and prescription drugs can all alter brain function.
- Consume good fats (omega-3 fatty acids) – These are needed for actual brain tissue and anti-inflammation from green vegetables, sea algae and vegetables, nuts, seeds, fish, and supplements.
- Get daily sunshine (fifteen to twenty minutes) – This is important for mood enhancement and vitamin D synthesis. Consider using a morning light box. Take 2000 to 5000 IU of vitamin D.
- Get daily exercise (thirty to sixty minutes) – Exercise is a mood elevator and improves blood flow to the brain.
- Get a good night's sleep – This helps with stress reduction, reducing stress hormones, and improves tissue repair.

Training Your Mind as You Would Train Your Body

One of my favorite quotes to share with patients is to *"train your mind as you would train your body for a marathon. Do it daily with intention."*

Think of your mind as a muscle that needs training. Expect to train it for two to three months before you really start to see change. Commit to a program for six months to a year. That is why I use the marathon analogy: You can't train for a marathon in a week. It takes months of hard work. Set a plan to train your mind in whatever discipline or disciplines feel right for you.

I believe it is critically important to do three things for your mind/spirit training on a daily basis:

1. Be quiet daily for fifteen to sixty minutes.
2. Be thankful morning and evening.
3. Hold a vision of what you want for your body and your life.

And truthfully, there is probably a fourth: Read or listen to positive things daily.

(Step 7) BE Thankful for Five Minutes Morning and Evening

Being thankful is an incredibly important and simple mental state of intention we can do to create a happy life, good health, and make the world a better place to live. Being continually thankful and living thankfully acknowledges and puts faith into action that there is a loving God or universal power.

Some of the "magic" that comes from being thankful is that if your mind is full of thankfulness there is no room for negative thinking. You don't have to try not to have negative thoughts; there just is no space for them in the thankful mind! Some believe that by the "Law of Attraction" you receive more of what you are thankful for. Since being thankful is a happier way to live than being negative, you have nothing to lose by practicing thankfulness and wonderful things to gain.

Start by just committing to being thankful for a few minutes every morning and evening. Then expand this thankfulness throughout your day. It's a wonderful way to live and will improve your physical and emotional health. Another way of saying this is *living in a state of gratitude.*

(Step 8) SIT Quietly for
Fifteen to Sixty Minutes Daily

Any type of meditative time—whether it's a traditional meditative practice or a prayer session, walking on the beach, or just sitting—is a critical component to being well.

Modern society provides so much for us to do that our minds find it difficult to be "empty" to receive or "hear" guidance from within.

For me, a transformational practice for the last couple of years has been just sitting still for fifteen to thirty minutes each day—physically still. I don't try to meditate or empty my mind of thoughts; I just accept the thoughts that come and don't worry about them. In the past when I tried to meditate, I always felt I failed. I would have so many thoughts in my mind and would "fight" to get them out of my mind.

Try just being physically still for fifteen to thirty minutes each day, in the same location, without worrying about your thoughts. It sounds simple, but practicing this every day has changed my life. Before I sit, I do one thing: I ask to *see my next step* clearly when I come out of my quiet time—the next step to really living my life's purpose, passion, and potential. If I have the quiet time, I usually see the next step and recognize it sometime later in the day or the next day.

(Step 9) IMAGINE Your Ideal Health and
Life Daily for Five to Fifteen Minutes.

Think about what you want, not about what
you don't want. Write it down. Picture it!

One thing I have noticed over the years is that chronically ill patients have no idea of what it's like to be well. If you ask them to picture themselves well or living their ideal life, many times they have no idea of what that might be. They can't even begin to imagine or describe it.

We create our reality first in our minds. What we think we become. The magic of picturing yourself well keeps you from thinking the worst about yourself, which strips you of hope. If nothing else, visualizing ourselves being well keeps us from focusing on being sick and all our problems, which doesn't help anyone.

One of the most important things you can do is just sit and imagine yourself in a perfect state of well-being—*whatever that means to you*. The other image is picturing your ideal life: what it is that you really want to do each and every moment. What excites you?

I call this practice of doing, visualizing, and speaking about what you really want to do with your life "giving your body the live message!" However you can give your body the live message is very important for living a truly healthy life. For me, it's living my life's work and being successful at it: teaching, writing, and encouraging people how to be and stay well and to live their life's passion. That is my joy and purpose. When I am living this, I feel whole, vibrant, and alive. When I am struggling with this, I don't feel well. In my most frustrating times, when that goal seemed farthest away, I felt as if I was dying.

Creating Your "Ideal Health Scene"

In his fabulous book (which has a two-CD audio version) *The Greatest Secret of All: Moving Beyond Abundance to a Life of True Fulfillment* (New World Library, 2008; NewWorldLibrary.com), Marc Allen proposes a fantastically simple, easy, and organized way of getting what you want in life.[1]

There's no reason why this process can't apply to other aspects of your life, such as your health goals. The following is my modification of Marc Allen's concept directed toward personal health.

1. Write down on one or two sheets of paper what your ideal "health scene" five years from now would be. Don't think too much. Just write down exactly how you would like your health and physical appearance to be. Do not let your mind

talk you out of picturing anything you want to be or look like. Just write it down.

2. Look at your perfect "health scene," see what health goals are present there, and write down your goals on a piece of paper.

3. Take each goal and write a positive affirmation about it. Allen has a unique way of prefacing any affirmation: "In an easy and relaxed manner and in a healthy and positive way..." You may end your affirmation by saying "...For this I am now so thankful and grateful," or in whatever way resonates with you.

4. Sit quietly and imagine your perfect health for five minutes daily. Imagine yourself being, doing, feeling, and radiating great health, doing the things you love to do each day.

5. Now take each of your health goals and write a plan for it. Take a step on each plan each week. Periodically review your plans and adjust accordingly.

Creating a Life Purpose Statement

I encourage everyone to try this simple "Life Purpose Exercise" by answering the following four questions that lead you to your "Life Purpose Statement." I believe a very important aspect of being healthy is living your *life's purpose.*[2]

1. List two of your unique personal qualities, such as *enthusiasm* and *creativity*.

2. List one or two ways you enjoy expressing those qualities when interacting with others, such as to *support* and *inspire*.

3. Assume the world is perfect right now. What does this world look like? How is everyone interacting with everyone else? What does it feel like? Write your answer as a statement, in the present tense, describing the ultimate condition, the perfect world as you see it and feel it. Remember: A perfect world is a fun place to be.

4. Combine the three prior subdivisions of this paragraph into a single statement.

This "Life Purpose Exercise" comes from Jack Canfield's excellent book *The Success Principles: How to Get From Where You Are to Where You Want to Be.* Canfield gives credit for learning this version of this "Life Purpose Exercise" to Arnold M. Patent, author of *You Can Have it All* and *The Journey* (Arnoldpatent.com). I say "thank you" to both of them. This simple exercise has been a catapult for me in getting on track with my life.

Here's my "Life's Purpose Statement," which I created within the last three years (I am a late bloomer!):

> "I, Kirkham Hamilton, use my energy and honesty to teach and inspire the people of the world to be confidently healthy, and to joyfully encourage individuals to follow their life's passions to the fullest, while they encourage others to do the same in a spirit of peace, joy, respect, and cooperation between people, animals, and the environment."

It's an interesting thing how the universe works, always giving you what you need to take the next step if you are open and receiving. I was listening to and reading a lot of Jack Canfield's work, as his way of presenting material resonated with me. I was in a bookstore looking for something else when *Success Principles* caught my eye. I liked Jack Canfield, so I bought the book even though I wasn't looking for it. I took it home with the intention of reading the whole thing—all 473 pages! To make a long story short, I never got past page twenty-three of the book, where the "Life Purpose Exercise" was—and I don't believe I was supposed to. God gave me that book to get the information on page twenty-three so I could focus my life more on achieving my dreams.

Several months later, I was in the same bookstore looking for a Jack Canfield audio CD series I really liked called *Maximum Confidence.* I couldn't find it, but right next to where I was looking was the Marc Allen audio CD set of *The Greatest Secret of All.* It just jumped out at me. It looked interesting, and it was only two CDs, so I knew no matter what I could get through them. Bingo! Those two CDs by Marc Allen changed my life. They were exactly what I needed: short, simple, to the point, and practical. I was looking to simplify all this self-improvement stuff I was working on, and Marc Allen made it *so* simple! It was perfect for me to "laser down" my focus on my dreams, goals, and plans, which seemed to be scattered all over the place.

I devoured that two-CD set about twenty times, and then one day I played hooky from a medical seminar in San Diego. I drove to the beach, sat in a little coffee shop, and two hours later had written my "five-year ideal scene" down to precise detail on just two pages. That was twenty-five years of scattered goals and dreams consolidated and refined. The point is this: I had been asking with all my heart for the last four or five years to really get my life's path together. Maybe it was turning fifty—who knows?—but I just felt it was my time to really share my gifts and that I'd better get my act together. Again, God sent me what I needed at the right time. God is perfect. Always offering the *next step*—if you ask and are open to receiving.

The works of these two wonderful teachers (Canfield and Allen) came at the exact right time. I was more ready. My focus was and is better. Most importantly, my quiet time is better, so I can "see" (hear) the messages God is giving me quicker and more clearly, and I have more confidence that I am being led.

Some Thoughts on the Validity of Imagery

Some might say that this imagery and picturing what you want is all "hocus pocus." A little too "out there." Yet most everyone accepts the use of imagery in athletics as normal. Many great athletes do it. During the Beijing Olympics in 2008 and the Vancouver Olympics in 2010, you probably heard more than one athlete say they pictured or visualized winning the race or their event over and over to perfection in their minds. Then it happened. Almost exactly as they imagined. Maybe even better!

If you believe imagery can be used for athletic performance, then it is not a far-fetched notion to believe that imagery can help us achieve a state of wellness with the physical body and abilities we want. Visualizing can't hurt and takes very little time. Just thinking about yourself being whole and vibrant has to create something positive physically instead of living in fear that your body is "falling apart."

If nothing else, thinking and imagining your ideal health state leaves no room in your mind for negative imagery.

These practices in the **TRIAD Mind-Body** section are not mine. They are from others with my own little twist and stories. Ultimately, if they resonate with you, they are really from God, lovingly guiding you to take the next step to fulfilling your true passions and walking your path on this planet, which is true health—to be able to live your life purpose with vibrancy, energy, passion, compassion, and most importantly love! Why else be healthy?

True Healing

I believe your mind leads your body. It is the master. That said, any way you get positive momentum going or tighten a few spokes, whether you start with your mind first or physical changes from diet and exercise, moving positively is the key. Ideally, you do it all at once, tightening a couple of mental and physical spokes at the same time. You marry positive mental practices with good lifestyle practices, and wonderful things happen! I guarantee it!

Conclusion
REMEMBER HOW WE GOT HERE

Modern humans, as they move from rural areas to cities (urbanization), have more access to excess calories and fewer nutrients from the increased consumption of processed foods. These changes in dietary intake have been facilitated by improvements in worldwide transportation, marketing, and manufacturing. In addition, people are less physically active in their daily jobs and getting to those jobs. These modern lifestyle factors lead to unhealthy weight gain and body inflammation that initiate and propagate all chronic diseases (i.e., heart disease, stroke, high blood pressure, cancer, diabetes, bone loss, Alzheimer's and Parkinson's diseases, macular degeneration, cataracts, etc.).

Medical research over the last thirty to forty years has shown that we can reverse chronic diseases, such as heart disease and diabetes, with *simple but aggressive* lifestyle practices involving diet and exercise. If done with consistency, lifestyle changes by far exceed anything that medication, hormones, or nutritional supplements can do for chronic disease management.

We have been afraid to use the word *"reverse"* for the major killers such as heart disease, diabetes, and obesity. This is wrong. These diseases can be reversed with very low-cost, low-technology approaches, and minimal medical resources—*but you have to be educated, you have to choose, you have to be committed, and you have to act!* Other chronic diseases—such as cancer, hypertension, stroke, bone loss, bone fractures, and degenerative eye and brain disorders—can be dramatically reduced or delayed and, in some cases, reversed as well.

Real Healthcare Reform

There is intense debate about how to improve healthcare efficiency, cover all Americans, and put some real prevention into our present disease-care model of healthcare. The problem I see is too many compromises with industries and institutions that have to be drastically changed if we are to be a truly healthy society. The whole medical industrial complex has to be downsized, and the pharmaceutical industry must become a second or third option to medical treatment, not the primary approach. Industries that produce unhealthy, highly processed foods and not whole, healthy foods will have to become much smaller. I don't want these changes occurring from government mandate, but from smart and educated consumers. If we simply make good choices with the food we eat and practice these *9 Simple Steps to Optimal Health,* we will change these industries and institutions literally overnight without "firing a shot!" *I envision educated consumers who understand that what they put in their mouths, how they move their bodies, and how they think are the most powerful medicines.* If the government does anything, I want them to disseminate good, credible health information and give economic incentives to individuals, businesses, and industries that help us *stay well* and *use fewer* medical services. Not pay more and more for disease care.

I hope you can see that through your understanding of the problem of disease care and chronic diseases, and living the lifestyle practices it takes to prevent and reverse most of these conditions, this is the greatest healthcare reform possible. **Real healthcare reform is totally in your hands now that you are educated.** *Don't blame your government, doctor, employer, or your union. Look at yourself in the mirror. That's who is responsible for your health. You have to get off your behind and go do it, and healthcare reform is a moot issue!*

Good Health is Achievable for You, Our Country, the World

If I have imparted anything in this book, it is the belief that you can improve your health—*right now!*—and that good health for most everyone is not a mystery. It is harder to be a single mom of three kids, start a new business, take care of an ailing or aging family member or spouse, or figure out the stock market.

For almost all of us, plugging your body into the **TRIAD Wellness Program's** *9 Simple Steps to Optimal Health* (three phases, with three steps to each phase) is a simple formula that is guaranteed to produce improved health. Good things will happen—and they can happen very quickly!

My hope is that by now you believe you can live in a world where people are healthy and all people are living their passion and sharing their gifts with the world. The planet is big enough for all of us. It's simple, and it does get fun. I promise!

My Last Pitch

There are two bold sections of my "Life Purpose Statement" that I truly wish for all of you:

> "I, Kirkham Hamilton, use my energy and honesty to teach and inspire **the people of the world to be confidently healthy** and to joyfully encourage **individuals to follow their life's passions to the fullest**, while they encourage others to do the same in a spirit of peace, joy, respect, and cooperation between people, animals, and the environment."

My patients and those who see me speak sometimes don't understand. I see them well. I can picture it clearly. I can see them doing it. I know they can do it! I realize that sometimes my belief in them is stronger than their belief in themselves. Sometimes my enthusiasm and challenge to them can be misunderstood as cocky, pushy, hard, not compassionate, or just plain overwhelming. But

I think most of my patients—not all—know how much I love and care about them and *want them to be in charge of their own health.*

Lastly, when I look at you, the reader, I see you well and vibrant. I see you right now stronger, more energetic, spending more time doing what you love to do, and fired up and confident that you can do this. I see you practicing these simple principles. From the depth of my total being, in the words of my ever-present and beloved mother, I say to you, *"You can do it!"*

Until the next time, *Be* and *Stay Well!*

9 Simple Steps to Optimal Health

TRIAD Wellness Program

3 Phases x 3 Steps

I. TRIAD Diet Program:

1. **EAT whole, unprocessed foods** (90 percent or more as plant foods, if not all plant foods).
2. **EAT** at least half your food intake as **vegetables**.
3. **ELIMINATE** all **dairy products** or eat from the **Basic Elimination Diet (BED)** for at least one month.

II. TRIAD Exercise Program:

4. **DO** a half-hour minimum of daily **aerobic exercise**.
5. **DO strength training** (circuit training) fifteen to thirty minutes, three to four days per week.
6. **DO flexibility training** (tai chi, yoga, Pilates, stretching) ten to sixty minutes daily.

III. TRIAD Mind-Body:

7. **BE thankful** for five minutes, morning and evening.
8. **SIT quietly** for fifteen to sixty minutes daily.
9. **IMAGINE your ideal health** and life daily for five to fifteen minutes. Think about what you want, not about what you don't want. Write it down. Picture it!

Appendix A

Basic Elimination Diet (BED)

- If on a whole-food, unrefined-food, vegetable-based diet you still feel poorly, *food intolerance* may be an issue.
- Write down foods you normally eat for four to seven days on the Diet-Exercise-Symptom Diary (see PDF printout at Prescription2000.com under Educational Handouts).
- Eat off the BED list of foods for at least two weeks (preferably four weeks). If there is a food on the BED list that you normally eat four or more times per week, eliminate it also.
- All your food should be whole food and half or more of your food intake should be vegetables off the BED list.
- After at least two and preferably four weeks, reintroduce the previous most commonly eaten foods one at a time for two days. Note symptoms. If tolerated, go to the next previous most commonly eaten food. You may re-introduce reactive foods into your diet after one month on a non-daily basis (every three to four days). If tolerated, keep it in the diet on a rotational basis. If reactive, eliminate it for six months, and then try again.
- If you still feel after one month that you have food-intolerant symptoms, you may need to get food intolerance/allergy testing; eat off a blood-type food list; do a comprehensive stool analysis; take pre- or probiotic supplementation; improve digestion; and/or see a physician competent in dealing with food intolerance.

Basic Elimination Diet Shopping List

Vegetables
Alfalfa Sprouts
Artichoke
Asparagus
Avocado
Beets
Bok Choy
Broccoli
Brussels Sprout
Cabbage
Carrots
Cauliflower
Celery
Chard
Collard Greens
Cucumber
Daikon Radish
Endive
Escarole
Green or Yellow (Beans)
Jicama
Kale
Kelp
Kohlrabi
Leeks
Lettuce
Mushrooms
Mustard Greens
Okra
Onions
Parsnips
Radishes
Rutabaga
Seaweed

Snow Peas
Spinach
Squash
Sweet Potato
Swiss Chard
Taro
Turnips
Water Chestnuts
Yams
Zucchini

Fruit
Apples
Apricots
Banana
Blackberries
Blueberries
Grapes
Kiwi
Mango
Melon
Nectarine
Papaya
Peaches
Pears
Pineapple
Plums
Pomegranate
Prunes
Raspberries
Strawberries
Watermelon

Beans/Legumes
Dried Beans
Dried Peas
Edamame
Lentils
Miso
Soy Milk
Tempeh
Tofu (Soy Bean)

Grains
Amaranth
Buckwheat
Millet
Cream of Rice
Puffed Rice
Rice Brown
Rice Bread
Rice Cakes (plain)
Rice Cereals (plain)
Rice Milk
Rice Pasta
Rice White
Quinoa

Nuts and Seeds
Almonds
Almond Milk
Flaxseeds
Hazelnuts
Pecans
Pumpkin Seeds
Sesame Seeds
Sunflower Seeds
Walnuts

Animal Foods (optional)
Beef
Chicken
Lamb
Pork
Poultry
Turkey
Wild Game
Cod
Halibut
Mackerel
Salmon
Sole
Trout
Tuna

Types of Elimination Diets

1. Basic Elimination Diet (BED). Eat off this list only (allows for all food groups except dairy). Eat unprocessed food only. Half your food intake *or more* is vegetables.

2. BED food list minus beef, grains, and soy/tofu (allows for all food groups except dairy, beef, soy, and grains). Eat unprocessed food only. Half your food intake *or more* is vegetables.

3. BED food list minus legumes and grains (allows for animal protein, nuts, seeds, vegetables, and fruit only). Eat unprocessed food only. Half your food intake *or more* is vegetables.

4. BED food list minus animal protein, grains, nuts, and seeds (allows for beans/legumes, fruit, and vegetables only). "Bean & Green Diet." Eat unprocessed food only. Half your food intake *or more* is vegetables.

5. BED food list minus animal protein, grains, beans/legumes, nuts, and seeds (allows for fruit and vegetables only). Eat unprocessed food only. Half your food intake *or more* is vegetables. (**Note:** This food list is a maximal anti-inflammatory diet. Get clearance from your physician before beginning this restricted diet for one to four weeks.)

Appendix B

Anti-Inflammatory Diet Principles

An anti-inflammatory diet is generally low in meat, egg, and dairy fat (unless these animals are free-ranged, antibiotic and hormone free, and eating omega-3-rich plants or are wild game), trans-fats (hydrogenated vegetable oils), and common food allergens, while high in antioxidants and phytonutrients generally from vegetables and fruit and, to a lesser extent, nuts, seeds, and whole grains. (Sometimes only non-glutinous grains are tolerated, necessitating eliminating wheat, oat, barley, and rye.)

Adding fish or fish oils, or omega-3 rich sea vegetables or algae-derived fatty acids can produce prostaglandins that have an anti-inflammatory effect. An anti-inflammatory effect can also occur using specific omega-6 fatty acids (GLA and DGLA) that come from borage and primrose oil as well. Though not as "popular" as omega-3 fatty acid rich fish oils, primrose oil or borage oil can provide significant anti-inflammatory effects.

Flaxseed oil is an omega-3 fat that comes from plants and can be converted, though in humans this is not efficiently done, into anti-inflammatory prostaglandins. Getting the oil from grinding fresh flaxseed is the preferred way to consume flaxseed oil. Flaxseeds may have anti-inflammatory effects in their own right. Ground flaxseed also contains other compounds that are beneficial, including lignans. Green, leafy plant foods are also a source of omega-3 fatty acids and in general is very beneficial because green leafy vegetables are the most nutrient-dense food available for mass consumption, with concentrated antioxidants, vitamins, minerals, phytonutrients, compounds, and protein (yes, protein!).

Sea vegetation (algae) and seaweed rich in omega-3 fatty acids are also rich in trace minerals and are anti-inflammatory. Sea vegetables are rich in iodine, which is good for your thyroid and, possibly more important, may help detoxify (compete with) compounds such as chlorine, bromine, and fluoride that may be harmful to the body.

The basic elimination diet (BED; Appendix A) is an excellent anti-inflammatory diet if whole foods and only the vegetables, fruit, whole grains (non-glutinous), beans, nuts, seeds, and fish off the list are eaten. In fact, the completely vegetarian version of this diet has been used in trials treating rheumatoid arthritis with success.[1]

Anti-Inflammatory Diets: What are the Components?

The following is a list of components of anti-inflammatory diets taken from medical studies that describe diets used to treat very serious inflammatory disorders, such as rheumatoid arthritis, lupus erythematosus, and other autoimmune disorders.[2] These same components of anti-inflammatory diets can reduce the incidence of all the chronic diseases of modern, industrialized societies caused by excess inflammation.

- Only whole, non-processed foods are consumed
- Reduced arachidonic acid (a pro-inflammatory fatty acid in excessive or imbalanced amounts) predominantly from meat, egg, and dairy fat
- Food elimination of "common allergens"
- Gluten- and dairy-free diets
- Vegan diet (no animal products) and gluten-free (no wheat, oat, barley, rye, couscous, etc.)
- Fish consumption, especially cold-water fish, if animal foods are consumed
- Nutrient supplementation used in some of these studies: vitamins C, D, E, B12, selenium, fish, flax, and/or bean oils (Note: Additional anti-inflammatory nutrients not used in

these studies: vitamin E with mixed tocopherols and tocotrienols, beta carotene with mixed carotenoids, magnesium, N-acetylcysteine, alpha lipoic acid, coenzyme Q10, MSM, glucosamine HCL, pycnogenol, resveratrol, ginger and tumeric, pomegranate, and concord grape juice, etc.)

Fasting: The Ultimate Anti-Inflammatory Diet

Fasting is the ultimate anti-inflammatory diet. It allows your immune system and gastrointestinal tract to "rest." When this occurs, inflammation is dramatically reduced and many body complaints disappear. There may be some elimination of toxins. Many times, there is a dramatic reversal of chronic disease.

Your G.I. tract is the largest surface area in your body and has an immune system all its own called GALT (gut activated lymphoid tissue). With chronic immune activation, inflammatory chemicals are released that can cause pain, swelling, and irritation anywhere in the body—*anywhere!* If this G.I. surface becomes more porous, the medical term is "increased intestinal permeability." Things that would normally *not* get absorbed do, because you have bigger (microscopic) holes in your gut that allow all kinds of substances from your gut—such as bacteria, fungi, partially digested food particles, toxic metabolites from bacteria, and fungi-eating undigested food that come into the bowel and other metabolites (organic acids)—to be reabsorbed into your circulation and cause problems anywhere in your body, not just in your gut. These problems can include headaches, joint and muscle pain, lethargy, foggy thinking, etc. Some of these same metabolites can be measured in a sophisticated test for body biochemistry called an *organic acid test.* A morning urine test for organic acids done by an experienced lab (Metametrix, Genova Diagnostics, Doctor's Data, or Great Plains Laboratories; see Resources and Organizations) can give a wealth of information regarding true body biochemistry.

There are many serious inflammatory or autoimmune conditions that, with appropriate implementation of fasting with water, juice, vegetable broth, or even just an intake of only fruit, vegetables, and water, can result in profound improvement in very serious conditions. Water, juice, or vegetable broth-only diets, as well as eating only fruit and vegetables, while generally very safe in the short term, should have the approval, knowledge, and oversight of a physician. If this is not possible, you can find a fasting-knowledgeable physician by contacting the International Association of Hygienic Physicians (iahp.net). This is a professional association for licensed, primary care physicians—medical doctors, osteopaths, chiropractors, and naturopaths—who specialize in therapeutic fasting supervision. A very experienced group of health professionals that do medically supervised fasting is True NorthHealth Center, in Santa Rosa, California (healthpromoting.com).

An excellent example of the incredible anti-inflammatory power of fasting is shown in this review paper of six cases of severe autoimmune diseases (rheumatoid arthritis, systemic lupus erythematosus, fibromyalgia, mixed connective tissue disease) where subjects underwent seven to twenty-four days of water fasting with *dramatic reductions in symptoms* plus outstanding weight loss. The individuals were then re-introduced to a carefully designed vegan diet to maintain symptom relief.[3]

Water Fasting Weight-Loss Results

Case 1: Rheumatoid arthritis—61-year-old male—18.5 pounds lost in 17 days

Case 2: Mixed connective tissue disease—38-year-old female—20.5 pounds lost in 21 days

Case 3: Fibromyalgia—46-year-old female—20.5 pounds lost in 24 days

Case 4: Systemic lupus erytheatosus—45-year-old female—8.4 pounds lost in 7 days

Case 5: Rheumatoid arthritis—40-year-old female—15 pounds lost in 12 days

Case 6: Rheumatoid arthritis—46-year-old female—49 pounds lost in 24 days

The foods we eat are the major triggers of inflammation, which leads to chronic or severe disease over time. We can reverse this excess inflammation that causes disease by changing to an anti-inflammatory diet (and lifestyle).

Resources and Organizations

Age Wave (agewave.com)
- Forward-thinking educational company on population aging and its profound business, social, healthcare, financial, workforce, and cultural implications.

Ani Phyo (aniphyo.com)
- Delicious, simple, organic, and fast whole food recipes.

American College for Advancement in Medicine (acam.org)
- Physicians practicing nutrition and integrative medicine.

Celiac Disease Foundation (celiac.org)
- Nonprofit providing services and support regarding celiac disease and dermatitis herpetiformis.

Doctor's Data Laboratory (doctorsdata.com)
- Specializing in the assessment, detection, prevention, and treatment of heavy metal burden, nutritional deficiencies, gastrointestinal function, hepatic detoxification, metabolic abnormalities, and diseases of environmental origin.

Genova Diagnostics Laboratory (genovadiagnostics.com)
- Functional laboratory testing focused on wellness and prevention to identify problems before chronic conditions and diseases develop. Specializing in comprehensive panels that combine standard and innovative biomarkers to provide a more complete understanding of specific biological systems.

Grass Roots Health (grassrootshealth.net)
- A public health promotion consortium of scientists, institutions, and individuals committed to solving the worldwide vitamin D deficiency epidemic.

Great Plains Laboratory (greatplainslaboratory.com)
- Provides testing for nutritional factors in chronic illnesses such as fibromyalgia, autism, and ADD, including immune deficiency evaluation, amino acid, essential fatty acid and organic acid testing, glutathione levels, metal toxicity, and food allergies tests.

International Association of Hygienic Physicians (iahp.net)
- A professional association for licensed primary care physicians who specialize in therapeutic fasting supervision.

International Water and Health Alliances (info@waterinternational.org)
- Nonprofit organization committed to disseminating information on water testing and solar pasteurization efforts worldwide to reduce water-borne disease, a major cause of hospitalizations and healthcare expenditures in developing countries.

Metametrix Clinical Laboratory (metametrix.com)
- A worldwide clinical laboratory specializing in the testing of nutrients, toxicants, hormonal balance, biotransformation and detoxification, gastrointestinal function, and the microbiome, assisting physicians in the prevention, mitigation, and treatment of complex chronic disease.

National Allergy Supply (natlallergy.com)
- Allergy supplies to control the home environment.

NY Coalition for Healthy School Food (healthyschoolfood.org)
- Nonprofit that works to improve the health and well-being of students by advocating for healthy plant-based foods, local and organic when possible, farm to school programs, school gardens, the elimination of unhealthy competitive foods in all areas of the school, comprehensive nutrition policy, and education to create food- and health-literate students.

Physicians Committee for Responsible Medicine (pcrm.org)

- A nonprofit organization that promotes preventive medicine, plant-based diets; conducts clinical research on chronic disease; and encourages higher standards for ethics and effectiveness in research.

Prescription 2000 Inc. (prescription2000.com)

- A health education company focused on disseminating credible research on chronic disease prevention and reversal for the public and professionals through print and audio interviews, health letters, books, webinars, public speaking, and other educational resources.

Prostate Cancer Research Institute (PCRI.org)

- A nonprofit organization committed to educating the public and professionals on prostate cancer prevention, detection, and treatment with an emphasis on active surveillance and using the most current but least invasive medical therapies that preserve the integrity of the body and dignity of the individual.

Solar Cookers International (solarcookers.org)

- A nonprofit spreading solar cooking awareness and skills worldwide. Founded in 1987, SCI has enabled over 30,000 families in Africa to cook with the sun's energy.

T. Colin Campbell Foundation (tcolincampbell.org)

- Nonprofit providing scientific research for the public and health professionals on the role of whole-foods and plant-based diets in preventing and reversing chronic disease.

The Blue Zones (bluezones.com)

- Provides scientific evidence from around the world on credible longevity research by studying documented healthy aging populations (Blue Zones) where people reach age 100 at rates 10 times greater than in the United States: suffer a fraction of the rate of heart disease and cancer, and where people live an extra 10 years compared to the United States.

The Cancer Project (cancerproject.org)

- Advances cancer prevention and survival through nutrition education and research, providing classes, books, video programs, fact sheets, brochures, and other educational materials.

The Okinawa Program and Diet (okinawaprogram.com)

- Provides scientifically documented longevity information based on the 25-year Okinawa Centenarian Study on one of the healthiest and longest-lived populations in the world.

TrueNorth Health Center (healthpromoting.com)

- A health center focused on disease prevention and reversal using physician-supervised therapeutic fasting, if appropriate (greater than 7,000 supervised fasts), and nutrition education on whole-food, non-processed plant-based diets.

VegNews (vegnews.com)

- The premiere magazine for up-to-date information on living a vegetarian, compassionate, and healthy lifestyle.

Vitamin D Council (vitamindcouncil.org)

- Disseminates up-to-date scientific research on the importance of recognizing vitamin D deficiency and vitamin D's role in the prevention and treatment of common chronic diseases.

Vitasearch (vitasearch.com)

- Complementary nutrition research website for professionals and the public, providing free weekly nutrition research updates (*Weekly Updates*), researcher interviews (*Expert Interviews*), and a searchable nutrition-oriented database (*Clinical Pearls*) of more than 35,000 article summaries.

Recommended Reading

21-Day Weight Loss Kickstart: Boost Metabolism, Lower Cholesterol, and Dramatically Improve Your Health by Neal Barnard, MD (2011).

Ani's Raw Food Essentials by Ani Phyo (2010).

Beating the Food Giants by Paul Stitt (1982).

The Blue Zone: Lessons for Living Longer From the People Who've Lived the Longest by Dan Buettner (2008).

Breaking the Food Seduction: The Hidden Reasons Behind Food Cravings—and 7 Steps to End Them Naturally by Neal Barnard, MD (2003).

Breaking the Vicious Cycle: Intestinal Health Through Diet (The Autism Connection) by Elaine Gottschall, BA, MSc (2004).

Building Bone Vitality: A Revolutionary Diet Plan to Prevent Bone Loss and Reverse Osteoporosis—Without Dairy Foods, Calcium, Estrogen, or Drugs by Amy Joy Lanou, PhD, and Michael Castleman (2009).

The China Study: Startling Implications for Diet, Weight Loss and Long-Term Health by T. Colin Campbell, PhD, and Thomas M. Campbell, PhD (2006).

Diet For A New America: How Your Food Choices Affect Your Health, Happiness, and the Future of Life on Earth by John Robbins (1987).

Doctor Neal Barnard's Program for Reversing Diabetes: The Scientifically Proven System For Reversing Diabetes Without Drugs by Neal D. Barnard, MD (2007).

Eat to Live: The Revolutionary Formula for Fast and Sustained Weight Loss by Joel Fuhrman, MD (2011).

The Engine 2 Diet: The Texas Firefighter's 28-Day Save-Your-Life-Plan that Lowers Cholesterol and Burns Away the Pounds by Rip Esselstyn (2009).

Food Allergy Survival Guide: Surviving and Thriving with Food Allergies and Sensitivities by Vesanto Melina, MS, RD; Jo Stepaniak, MSEd; and Dina Aronson, MS, RD (2004).

Food and Behavior: A Natural Connection by Barbara Reed Stitt (2004).

The Food Revolution, How Your Diet Can Help Save Your Life and Our World by John Robbins (2001).

The Greatest Secret of All by Marc Allen (two-CD audio set; 2008).

Healthy at 100: The Scientifically Proven Secrets of the World's Healthiest and Longest-Lived Peoples by John Robbins (2007).

Jack Canfield's Key to Living the Law of Attraction: A Simple Guide to Creating the Life of Your Dreams by Jack Canfield and D.D. Watkins (2007).

The Jungle Effect: A Doctor Discovers the Healthiest Diets From Around the World—Why They Work and How to Bring Them Home by Daphne Miller, MD (2008).

Living With Joy; Keys To Personal Power and Spiritual Transformation by Sanaya Roman (1989).

The Longevity Diet: Discover Calorie Restriction—the Only Proven Way to Slow the Aging Process and Maintain Peak Vitality by Brian M. Delaney and Lisa Walford (2005).

Love Medicine and Miracles by Bernie Siegel, MD (1986).

The Okinawa Diet Plan: The Only Diet With 100 Years of Living Proof by Bradley J. Willcox, MD; D. Craig Willcox, PhD; and Makoto Suzuki, MD, PhD (2004).

The Okinawa Program: How the World's Longest-Lived People Achieve Everlasting Health—And How You Can Too by Bradley J. Willcox, MD; D. Craig Willcox, PhD; and Makoto Suzuki, MD, PhD (2001).

The Pleasure Trap by Alan Goldhamer, DC and Douglas J. Lisle, PhD (2003).

Prevent and Reverse Heart Disease: The Revolutionary, Scientifically Proven, Nutrition-Based Cure by Caldwell B. Esselstyn Jr., MD (2007).

The Relaxation and Stress Reduction Workbook by Martha Davis, Elizabeth Robbins Eshelman, and Matthew McKay (2008).

Reverse Heart Disease Now: Stop Deadly Cardiovascular Plaque Before It's Too Late by Stephen T. Sinatra, MD, and James C. Roberts, MD (2007).

Spiritual Growth: Being Your Higher Self by Sanaya Roman (1989).

Stop Inflammation Now!: A Step-By-Step Plan to Prevent, Treat, and Reverse Inflammation—The Leading Cause of Heart Disease and Related Conditions by Richard M. Fleming, MD (2004).

Stretching: 30th Anniversary Edition by Bob and Jean Anderson (2010).

The Success Principles: How to Get from Where You Are to Where You Want to Be by Jack Canfield (2007).

The Unhealthy Truth: How Our Food Is Making Us Sick and What We Can Do About It by Robyn O'Brien (2009).

Whitewash: The Disturbing Truth About Cow's Milk and Your Health by Joseph Keon (2010).

Educational Resources at
Prescription2000.com

A Health Education Company by Kirk Hamilton

Staying Healthy Today Interviews

Staying Healthy Today with Kirk Hamilton Health Letter

Expert Pearls – Potential therapies in nutritional medicine from *Expert Interviews*

Educational Handouts – Self-help material emphasizing nutrition, prevention, and self-care

Educational Links – Links to credible nutrition and prevention oriented websites with an emphasis on chronic disease prevention and reversal

Staying Healthy Today Seminar Series - chronic disease prevention and reversal

Join our FREE Health Letter *Today!*
at Prescription2000.com

Notes

Chapter 1
Urbanization, the Modern Lifestyle, and Chronic Disease

1. Jiaquan Xu among others, "Deaths: Final Data for 2007." *National Vital Statistics Report.* 58, no. 19 (May 20, 2010): 1, 5. Table B. *Percentage of total deaths, death rates, age-adjusted death rates for 2007, percentage in age-adjusted death rates in 2007 from 2006, and ratio age-adjusted death rates by race and sex for the 15 leading causes of death for the total population in 2007: United States.* http://www.cdc.gov/nchs/data/nvsr/nvsr58/nvsr58_19.pdf (accessed Feb. 12, 2011); *The Power of Prevention Chronic Disease . . . The Public Health Challenge of the 21st Century, 2009.* Department of Health and Human Services – USA, National Center For Chronic Disease Prevention and Health Promotion, Centers for Disease Control: 1. http://www.cdc.gov/chronicdisease/pdf/2009-Power-of-Prevention.pdf (accessed Feb. 12, 2011); *Ten Facts About Chronic Disease.* World Health Organization. http://www.who.int/features/factfiles/chp/01_en.html (accessed Feb. 12, 2011).

2. Gerard Anderson, "Chronic Conditions: Making the Case for Ongoing Care." Baltimore, MD: John Hopkins University; November, 2007: 16, 22, 25. http://www.fightchronicdisease.org/news/pfcd/documents/ChronicCareChartbook_FINAL.pdf (accessed Feb. 15, 2011) ; *The Power of Prevention Chronic Disease . . . The Public Health Challenge of the 21st Century, 2009*, Department of Health and Human Services – USA, National Center For Chronic Disease Prevention and Healthy Promotion, Centers for Disease Control: 1. http://www.cdc.gov/chronicdisease/pdf/2009-Power-of-Prevention.pdf (accessed Feb. 12, 2011).

3. J. Lazarou, B.H. Pomeranz, and P.N. Corey, "Incidence of Adverse Drug Reactions in Hospitalized Patients: A Meta-analysis of Prospective Studies." *JAMA.* 279, no. 15 (April 1998): 1200-5.

4. *U.S. Food Supply: Nutrients and Other Food Components, Per Capita Per Day.* USDA/Center for Nutrition Policy and Promotion, Feb. 27, 2009. Data are based on ERS estimates of per capita quantities of food available for consumption, on imputed consumption data for foods no longer reported by ERS, and on estimates from USDA's Center for Nutrition Pol-

icy and Promotion (CNPP) of quantities of produce from home gardens. http://www.ers.usda.gov/Data/FoodConsumption/NutrientAvailIndex. htm (spreadsheets, click on totals) (accessed Feb. 12, 2011).

5. Jean Buzby and Hodan Farah Wells, *Average Daily Per Capita Calories From the U.S. Food Availability, Adjusted for Spoilage and Other Waste.* United States Department of Agriculture, Economic Research Service. Data last updated Feb. 1, 2010. Note: Loss factors presented here are first estimates and are intended to serve as a starting point for additional research and discussion. Questions & suggestions: Contact Jean Buzby at jbuzby@ers.usda.gov or Hodan Farah Wells at hfarah@ers.usda.gov. http://www.ers.usda.gov/Data/FoodConsumption/FoodGuideSpread-sheets.htm#calories (accessed Feb. 12, 2011).

6. Hodan Farah Wells and Jean Buzby, *Meat Consumption Patterns in the United States Over the Last 100 Years.* Source: USDA, Economic Research Service, Food Availability Data. Hodan Farah Wells, Ph.D., economist with the Economic Research Service, 1800 M Street NW, Washington, DC 20036, Phone: 202-694-5578, Fax: 202-694-5688, Email: hfarah@ers.usda.gov, Jean Buzby, Ph.D., agricultural economist with the Economic Research Service, Room S2080, 1800 M Street NW, Washington, DC 20036-5831. http://www.ers.usda.gov/Data/FoodConsumption/app/availability.aspx; http://www.ers.usda.gov/Data/FoodConsumption/app/loss_adjusted.aspx (accessed Feb. 12, 2011).

7. Hodan Farah Wells and Jean Buzby, *Fats and Oil Consumption Patterns in the United States Over the Last 100 Years.* USDA, Economic Research Service estimate using data from Census Bureau. Hodan Farah Wells, Ph.D., economist with the Economic Research Service, 1800 M Street NW, Washington, DC 20036, Phone: 202-694-5578, Fax: 202-694-5688, Email: hfarah@ers.usda.gov, Jean Buzby, Ph.D., agricultural economist with the Economic Research Service, Room S2080, 1800 M Street NW, Washington, DC 20036-5831. http://www.ers.usda.gov/Data/FoodConsumption/app/availability.aspx; http://www.ers.usda.gov/Data/FoodConsumption/app/loss_adjusted.aspx (accessed Feb. 12, 2011).

8. Hodan Farah Wells and Jean Buzby, *Calorie Sweetener Consumption Patterns in the United States Over the Last 100 Years.* Source: USDA, Economic Research Service, Food Availability Data. Hodan Farah Wells, Ph.D., economist with the Economic Research Service, 1800 M Street NW, Washington, DC 20036, Phone: 202-694-5578, Fax: 202-694-5688, Email: hfarah@ers.usda.gov, Jean Buzby, Ph.D., agricultural economist with the Economic Research Service, Room S2080, 1800 M Street NW, Washington, DC 20036-5831. http://www.ers.usda.gov/Data/FoodConsumption/app/availability.aspx; http://www.ers.usda.gov/Data/FoodConsumption/app/loss_adjusted.aspx (accessed Feb. 12, 2011).

9. Hodan Farah Wells and Jean Buzby, *Cheese Consumption Patterns in the United States Over the Last 100 Years.* Source: USDA, Economic Research Service, Food Availability Data. Hodan Farah Wells, Ph.D., economist with the Economic Research Service, 1800 M Street NW, Washington, DC 20036, Phone: 202-694-5578, Fax: 202-694-5688, Email: hfarah@ers.usda.gov, Jean Buzby, Ph.D., agricultural economist with the Economic Research Service, Room S2080, 1800 M Street NW, Washington, DC 20036-5831. http://www.ers.usda.gov/Data/FoodConsumption/app/availability.aspx; http://www.ers.usda.gov/Data/FoodConsumption/app/loss_adjusted. aspx (accessed Feb. 12, 2011).

10. Hodan Farah Wells and Jean Buzby, *Flour and Cereal Product Consumption Patterns in the United States Over The Last 100 Years.* Source: USDA, Economic Research Service, Food Availability Data. Hodan Farah Wells, Ph.D., economist with the Economic Research Service, 1800 M Street NW, Washington, DC 20036, Phone: 202-694-5578, Fax: 202-694-5688, Email: hfarah@ers.usda.gov, Jean Buzby, Ph.D., agricultural economist with the Economic Research Service, Room S2080, 1800 M Street NW, Washington, DC 20036-5831. http://www.ers.usda.gov/Data/FoodConsumption/FoodAvailSpreadsheets.htm#grains; http://www.ers.usda.gov/Data/FoodConsumption/app/availability.aspx; http://www.ers.usda.gov/Data/FoodConsumption/app/loss_adjusted.aspx (accessed February 12, 2011); Jean Buzby et al., "Will 2005 Be the Year of the Whole Grain?" *Amber Waves.* (June 2005). United States Department of Agriculture, Economic Research Service. http://www.ers.usda.gov/AmberWaves/June05/Features/Will2005WholeGrain.htm (accessed Feb. 12, 2011); Jean Buzby and Lisa Macino, "Americans' Whole-Grain Consumption Below Guidelines." *Amber Waves.* (April 2005): 5. United States Department of Agriculture, Economic Research Service. http://www.ers.usda.gov/Amberwaves/April05/Findings/WholeGrainConsumption.htm (accessed Feb. 12, 2011).

11. D.S. Ludwig and H.A. Pollack, "Obesity and the Economy: From Crisis to Opportunity." *JAMA.* 301, no. 5 (Feb. 4, 2009): 533–5.

12. *U.S. Food Consumption as a % of Calories,* New York Coalition for Healthy School Food, Copyright 2009. healthylunches.org. Special thanks to Amie Hamlin, Executive Director of *The New York Coalition for Healthy School Food* for permission to reproduce this chart. Source: USDA Economic Research Service, 2009; www.ers.usda.gov/publications/EIB33/; www.ers.usda.gov/Data/FoodConsumption/FoodGuideIndex.htm#calories Special thanks to Joel Fuhrman, MD, author of *Disease Proof Your Child: Feeding Kids Right* * Graphics by MichelleBando.com. http://www.healthyschoolfood.org/docs/color_pie_chart.pdf (accessed Feb. 12, 2011).

13. Stacey Rosen and Shahla Shapouri, "Obesity in the Midst of Unyielding Food Insecurity in Developing Countries." *Amber Waves.* (September 2008). http://www.ers.usda.gov/AmberWaves/September08/Features/ObesityCountries.htm (accessed Feb. 12, 2011).

Chapter 2
The American Lifestyle

1. Ken Dychtwald, *About Age Wave–A Visionary Company with Unparalleled Know-How About the Maturing Marketplace.* Age Wave website. http://www.agewave.com/about/index.php (accessed Feb. 12, 2011).

2. John Robbins, *Healthy at 100. How You Can–at Any Age–Dramatically Increase Your Life Span and Your Health Span* (New York: Random House, 2006), xv.

3. John Robbins, *Healthy at 100. How You Can–at Any Age–Dramatically Increase Your Life Span and Your Health Span* (New York: Random House, 2006), xvii.

4. Jiaquan Xu among others, "Deaths: Final Data for 2007." *National Vital Statistics Report.* 58, no. 19 (May 20, 2010): 1, 5. Table B. *Percentage of total deaths, death rates, age-adjusted death rates for 2007, percentage in age-adjusted death rates in 2007 from 2006, and ratio age-adjusted death rates by race and sex for the 15 leading causes of death for the total population in 2007: United States.* http://www.cdc.gov/nchs/data/nvsr/nvsr58/nvsr58_19.pdf (accessed Feb. 12, 2011); *The Power of Prevention Chronic Disease . . . The Public Health Challenge of the 21st Century, 2009.* Department of Health and Human Services – USA, National Center For Chronic Disease Prevention and Health Promotion, Centers for Disease Control: 1. http://www.cdc.gov/chronicdisease/pdf/2009-Power-of-Prevention.pdf (accessed Feb. 12, 2011).

5. B. Swinburn among others, "Increased Food Energy Supply is More Than Sufficient to Explain the US Epidemic of Obesity." *Am J Clin Nutr.* 90, no. 6 (Dec 2009): 1453–6. 2009 Oct. 14.

6. Jessica E. Todd and Lisa Mancino, "Eating Out Increases Daily Calorie Intake." *Amber Waves.* (June 2010). United States Department of Agriculture, Economic Research Service. http://www.ers.usda.gov/AmberWaves/June10/Findings/EatingOut.htm (accessed Feb. 12, 2011); Annette Clauson, *Food and Alcoholic Beverages: Total Expenditures.* Briefing Rooms: Food CPI and Expenditures: Table 1. United States Department of Agriculture, Economic Research Service. http://www.ers.usda.gov/Briefing/CPIFoodAndExpenditures/Data/Expenditures_tables/table1.htm (accessed Feb. 12, 2011).

7. Jessica E. Todd among others, "The Impact of Food Away From Home on Adult Diet Quality." *ERS Summary Report.* (February, 2010): 1. United States Department of Agriculture, Economic Research Service. http://www.ers.usda.gov/Publications/ERR90/ERR90_ReportSummary.pdf (accessed Feb. 12, 2011).

8. C.L. Ogden among others, "Prevalence of Overweight, Obesity, and Extreme Obesity Among Adults: United States, Trends 1976–1980 Through 2007–2008." (June 2010): 1, 5 (Table 1). National Center for Health Statistics. Centers for Disease Control and Prevention. http://www.cdc.gov/NCHS/data/hestat/obesity_adult_07_08/obesity_adult_07_08.pdf (accessed Feb. 12, 2011).

9. *Overweight and Obesity: Health Problems.* Centers for Disease Control and Prevention. http://www.cdc.gov/obesity/causes/health.html (accessed Feb. 12, 2011).

10. Cynthia Ogden and Margaret Carroll, *Prevalence of Obesity Among Children and Adolescents: United States, Trends 1963–1965 Through 2007–2008. Trends in Obesity Among Children and Adolescents: United States, 1963–2008* (Figure 1). *"Prevalence of Obesity Among U.S. Children and Adolescents Aged 2–19, For Selected Years 1963–1965 Through 2007–2008* (Table 1). Centers for Disease Control and Prevention. National Center for Health Statistics. http://www.cdc.gov/nchs/data/hestat/obesity_child_07_08/obesity_child_07_08.htm (accessed Feb. 12, 2011).

11. *Healthy Youth! Childhood Obesity.* National Center for Chronic Disease Prevention and Health Promotion. Centers for Disease Control and Prevention. http://www.cdc.gov/HealthyYouth/obesity/ (accessed Feb. 12, 2011).

12. S.J. Olshansky among others, "A Potential Decline in Life Expectancy in the United States in the 21st Century." *N Engl J Med.* 352, no. 11 (Mar. 17, 2005): 1138–45.

13. Hodan Farah Wells and Jean Buzby, *Meat Consumption Patterns in the United States Over the Last 100 Years.* Source: USDA, Economic Research Service, Food Availability Data. Hodan Farah Wells, Ph.D., economist with the Economic Research Service, 1800 M Street NW, Washington, DC 20036, Phone: 202-694-5578, Fax: 202-694-5688, Email: hfarah@ers.usda.gov, Jean Buzby, Ph.D., agricultural economist with the Economic Research Service, Room S2080, 1800 M Street NW, Washington, DC 20036-5831. http://www.ers.usda.gov/Data/FoodConsumption/app/availability. aspx ; http://www.ers.usda.gov/Data/FoodConsumption/app/loss_adjusted.aspx (accessed Feb. 12, 2011).

14. Hodan Farah Wells and Jean Buzby, *Fats and Oil Consumption Patterns in the United States Over the Last 100 Years.* USDA, Economic Research Service estimate using data from Census Bureau. Hodan Farah Wells, Ph.D., economist with the Economic Research Service, 1800 M Street NW, Washington, DC 20036, Phone: 202-694-5578, Fax: 202-694-5688, Email: hfarah@ers.usda.gov, Jean Buzby, Ph.D., agricultural economist with the Economic Research Service, Room S2080, 1800 M Street NW, Washington, DC 20036-5831. http://www.ers.usda.gov/Data/FoodConsumption/

app/availability.aspx; http://www.ers.usda.gov/Data/FoodConsumption/app/loss_adjusted.aspx (accessed Feb. 12, 2011).

15. Hodan Farah Wells and Jean Buzby, *Calorie Sweetener Consumption Patterns in the United States Over the Last 100 Years.* Source: USDA, Economic Research Service, Food Availability Data. Hodan Farah Wells, Ph.D., economist with the Economic Research Service, 1800 M Street NW, Washington, DC 20036, Phone: 202-694-5578, Fax: 202-694-5688, Email: hfarah@ers.usda.gov, Jean Buzby, Ph.D., agricultural economist with the Economic Research Service, Room S2080, 1800 M Street NW, Washington, DC 20036-5831. http://www.ers.usda.gov/Data/FoodConsumption/app/availability.aspx; http://www.ers.usda.gov/Data/FoodConsumption/app/loss_adjusted.aspx (accessed Feb. 12, 2011).

16. Hodan Farah Wells and Jean Buzby, *Cheese Consumption Patterns in the United States Over the Last 100 Years.* Source: USDA, Economic Research Service, Food Availability Data. Hodan Farah Wells, Ph.D., economist with the Economic Research Service, 1800 M Street NW, Washington, DC 20036, Phone: 202-694-5578, Fax: 202-694-5688, Email: hfarah@ers.usda.gov, Jean Buzby, Ph.D., agricultural economist with the Economic Research Service, Room S2080, 1800 M Street NW, Washington, DC 20036-5831. http://www.ers.usda.gov/Data/FoodConsumption/app/availability.aspx; http://www.ers.usda.gov/Data/FoodConsumption/app/loss_adjusted.aspx (accessed Feb. 12, 2011).

17. Hodan Farah Wells and Jean Buzby, *Flour and Cereal Product Consumption Patterns in the United States Over the Last 100 Years.* Source: USDA, Economic Research Service, Food Availability Data. Hodan Farah Wells, Ph.D., economist with the Economic Research Service, 1800 M Street NW, Washington, DC 20036, Phone: 202-694-5578, Fax: 202-694-5688, Email: hfarah@ers.usda.gov, Jean Buzby, Ph.D., agricultural economist with the Economic Research Service, Room S2080, 1800 M Street NW, Washington, DC 20036-5831. http://www.ers.usda.gov/Data/FoodConsumption/FoodAvailSpreadsheets.htm#grains; http://www.ers.usda.gov/Data/FoodConsumption/app/availability.aspx; http://www.ers.usda.gov/Data/FoodConsumption/app/loss_adjusted.aspx (accessed Feb. 12, 2011); Jean Buzby et al., "Will 2005 Be the Year of the Whole Grain?" *Amber Waves.* (June 2005). United States Department of Agriculture, Economic Research Service. http://www.ers.usda.gov/AmberWaves/June05/Features/Will2005WholeGrain.htm (accessed Feb. 12, 2011); Jean Buzby and Lisa Macino, "Americans' Whole-Grain Consumption Below Guidelines." *Amber Waves.* (April 2005): 5. United States Department of Agriculture, Economic Research Service. http://www.ers.usda.gov/Amberwaves/April05/Findings/WholeGrainConsumption.htm (accessed Feb. 12, 2011).

18. *Status of the Nation – A Need for Change: Adults – Adolescents and Young Adults – High School Students. Physical Activity and Healthy: A Report From the Surgeon General. At-A- Glance.* Centers for Disease Control and Preven-

tion, National Center for Chronic Disease Prevention and Health Promotion. http://www.cdc.gov/nccdphp/sgr/ataglan.htm (accessed Feb. 12, 2011).

19. *Inflammation.* Wikipedia, The Free Encyclopedia. http://en.wikipedia.org/wiki/Inflammation (accessed Jan. 29, 2011).

20. T. Edwards, "Inflammation, Pain, and Chronic Disease: An Integrative Approach to Treatment and Prevention." *Altern Ther Health Med.* 11, no. 6 (Nov.–Dec. 2005): 20–7; quiz 28, 75.

21. *Global Strategy on Diet, Physical Activity and Health. Facts Related to Chronic Diseases.* World Health Organization. http://www.who.int/hpr/gs.fs.chronic.disease.shtml#::%20FACTS;http://www.who.int/hpr/NPH/docs/gs_global_strategy_general.pdf (accessed Feb. 12, 2011).

Chapter 3:
Global Health: Where Are We Going?

1. *Ten Facts About Chronic Disease.* World Health Organization. http://www.who.int/features/factfiles/chp/01_en.html (accessed Feb. 13, 2011).

2. *Ten Facts About Chronic Disease.* World Health Organization. http://www.who.int/features/factfiles/chp/05_en.html (accessed Feb. 13, 2011).

3. *Ten Facts About Chronic Disease.* World Health Organization. http://www.who.int/features/factfiles/chp/10_en.html (accessed Feb. 13, 2011).

4. "Calorie Availability is Increasing in Developing Countries." *Amber Waves.* (September 2008). Source: Food and Agriculture Organization of the United Nations. United States Department of Agriculture, Economic Research Service. http://www.ers.usda.gov/AmberWaves/September08/Features/ObesityCountries.htm (accessed Feb. 13, 2011); "Grain Share of Developing Country Diet Shrinks...As Meat and Vegetable Oil Share Rise." *Amber Waves.* (September 2008). Source: Food and Agriculture Organization of the United Nations. United States Department of Agriculture, Economic Research Service. http://www.ers.usda.gov/AmberWaves/September08/Features/ObesityCountries.htm (accessed Feb. 13, 2011).

5. Stacey Rosen and Shahla Shapouri, "Obesity in the Midst of Unyielding Food Insecurity in Developing Countries." *Amber Waves.* (September 2008). http://www.ers.usda.gov/AmberWaves/September08/Features/ObesityCountries.htm (accessed Feb. 13, 2011).

6. *Obesity and Overweight: Facts About Overweight and Obesity.* World Health Organization, Media Centre, fact sheet no. 311, September 2006. http://www.who.int/mediacentre/factsheets/fs311/en/ (accessed Feb. 13, 2011).

7. *Obesity and Overweight: What Are Common Health Consequences of Overweight and Obesity?* World Health Organization, Media Centre, fact sheet no. 311, September 2006. http://www.who.int/mediacentre/factsheets/fs311/en/ (accessed Feb. 13, 2011).

8. *Obesity and Overweight: What Are Common Health Consequences of Overweight and Obesity?* World Health Organization, Media Centre, fact sheet no. 311, September 2006. http://www.who.int/mediacentre/factsheets/fs311/en/ (accessed Feb. 13, 2011).

9. *Obesity and Overweight: What Are Common Health Consequences of Overweight and Obesity?* World Health Organization, Media Centre, fact sheet no. 311, September 2006. http://www.who.int/mediacentre/factsheets/fs311/en/ (accessed Feb. 13, 2011).

10. Jane Parry, "China and Japan Face Epidemic of Heart Disease." *Br Med J.* 329, no. 7467 (Sept. 18, 2004): 643 doi: 10.1136/bmj.329.7467.643 (Published Sept. 16, 2004). http://www.bmj.com/content/329/7467/643.1.extract (accessed Feb. 13, 2011).

11. "India Overwhelmed by Heart Disease." *The China Post*, Updated Saturday, April 26, 2008 0:00 am TWN, AFP. http://www.chinapost.com.tw/health/heart/2008/04/26/153695/India-overwhelmedhtm (accessed Feb. 13, 2011).

12. *Cancer: Cancer Quick Facts.* World Health Organization. http://www.who.int/cancer/en/ (accessed Jan. 29, 2010); *Cancer: What Causes Cancer.* World Health Organization, Media Centre, fact sheet no. 297, February 2009. http://www.who.int/mediacentre/factsheets/fs297/en/index.html (accessed Feb. 13, 2011).

13. *Diabetes: Key Facts.* World Health Organization, Media Centre, fact sheet no. 312, November 2009. http://www.who.int/mediacentre/factsheets/fs312/en/; S. Wild and others, "Global Prevalence of Diabetes: Estimates for the Year 2000 and Projections for 2030." *Diabetes Care.* 27 (2004): 1047–1053. http://www.who.int/diabetes/facts/en/diabcare0504.pdf (accessed Feb. 13, 2011).

14. *Diabetes: What is Diabetes?* World Health Organization, Media Centre, fact sheet no.312, November 2009. http://www.who.int/mediacentre/factsheets/fs312/en/ (accessed Feb. 13, 2011).

15. *Diabetes: What is Diabetes?* World Health Organization, Media Centre, fact sheet no.312, November 2009. http://www.who.int/mediacentre/factsheets/fs312/en/ (accessed Feb. 13, 2011).

16. *Diabetes Basics: What is Gestational Diabetes?* American Diabetes Association. http://www.diabetes.org/diabetes-basics/gestational/what-is-gestational-diabetes.html (accessed Feb. 13, 2011).

17. *The Facts About Diabetes: America's Seventh Leading Cause of Death. How Many Americans Have Diabetes and Pre-Diabetes?* U.S. Department of Health and Human Services, National Diabetes Education Program. http://ndep.nih.gov/diabetes-facts/index.aspx (accessed Feb. 13, 2011).

18. *Diabetes: Quick Diabetes Facts.* World Health Organization, Diabetes Programme. http://www.who.int/diabetes/en/ (accessed Feb. 13, 2011).

19. *Cardiovascular Diseases (CVDs): Key Facts.* World Health Organization, Media Centre, fact sheet no.317, Updated September 2009. http://www.who.int/mediacentre/factsheets/fs317/en/index.html (accessed Feb. 13, 2011); *Global Causes of Death Move From Infectious to Chronic Diseases: Trend Due to Aging Populations in Middle-, Low-Income Nations, WHO Says.* America.Gov, June 12, 2008. http://www.america.gov/st/develop-english/2008/June/20080612141457lcnirellep0.7136347.html (accessed Feb. 13, 2011); World Health Organization, *World Health Statistics 2008.* (Geneva, Switzerland: WHO Press, 2008), 29. http://www.who.int/whosis/whostat/EN_WHS08_Full.pdf (accessed Jan. 29, 2011).

20. *Cardiovascular Diseases (CVDS): What Are the Risk Factors for Cardiovascular Disease?* World Health Organization, Media Centre, fact sheet no.317, Updated September 2009. http://www.who.int/mediacentre/factsheets/fs317/en/index.html (accessed Feb. 13, 2011).

21. *10 Facts on Ageing and the Life Course.* World Health Organization, September 2007. http://www.who.int/features/factfiles/ageing/en/index.html (accessed Feb. 13, 2011).

Chapter 4
Preventive Care vs. Disease Care: Changing the Paradigm

1. H.R. Ferdowsian , "A Multicomponent Intervention Reduces Body Weight and Cardiovascular Risk at a GEICO Corporate Site." *Am J Health Promot.* 24, no. 6 (July–Aug. 2010): 384–7.

Chapter 5
The Good News: Chronic Disease Is
Preventable and Reversible

1. *Obesity and Overweight: What Causes Obesity and Overweight?* World Health Organization, Media Centre, fact sheet no.311, September 2006. http://www.who.int/mediacentre/factsheets/fs311/en/index.html (accessed Feb. 13, 2011).

2. *Global Strategy on Diet, Physical Activity and Health: Diet.* World Health Organization. http://www.who.int/dietphysicalactivity/diet/en/index. html (accessed Feb. 13, 2011); Edward A. Fisher and others, "Summary of a Scientific Conference on Preventive Nutrition: Pediatrics to Geriatrics." Circulation. 100 (1999): 450–456. Also available from: http://circ. ahajournals.org/cgi/content/full/100/4/450#T1 and Table 3; http:// circ.ahajournals.org/cgi/content/full/100/4/450/T3 (accessed Jan. 29, 2011); "New Unified Dietary Guidelines Offer Nutritional Protection Against Wide Range Of Killer Diseases." *ScienceDaily.* (June 22, 1999). http://www.sciencedaily.com/releases/1999/06/990622061026.htm (accessed June 11, 2011).

3. *Global Strategy on Diet, Physical Activity and Health: Promoting Fruit and Vegetable Consumption Around the World – Introduction.* World Health Organization. http://www.who.int/dietphysicalactivity/fruit/en/index. html (accessed Feb. 13, 2011).

4. *Global Strategy on Diet, Physical Activity and Health: Diet and Physical Activity: A Public Health Priority.* World Health Organization. http://www. who.int/dietphysicalactivity/en/index.html (accessed Feb. 13, 2011).

5. *Cancer: How Can the Burden of Cancer Be Reduced?* World Health Organization. Media Centre. http://www.who.int/mediacentre/factsheets/ fs297/en/index.html (accessed Feb. 13, 2011); G. Danaei and others, "Causes Of Cancer In The World: Comparative Risk Assessment Of Nine Behavioural and Environmental Risk Factors." *Lancet.* 366, no. 9499 (November 2005): 1784–93.

6. *Skin Cancer Facts: General.* Skin Cancer Foundation. http://www.skincancer.org/Skin-Cancer-Facts/ (accessed Feb. 13, 2011).

7. *Skin Cancer Facts: Melanoma.* Skin Cancer Foundation. http://www.skin-cancer.org/Skin-Cancer-Facts/ (accessed Feb. 13, 2011).

8. P.N. Karnauchow, "Melanoma and Sun Exposure." *Lancet.* 346 (September 1995): 915. Vitasearch.com summary #23321. http://www.vitasearch. com/get-clp-summary/15511 (accessed Feb. 13, 2011); M.A. Weinstock and others, "Melanoma and The Sun: The Effect Of Swimsuits and A 'Healthy' Tan On The Risk of Nonfamilial Malignant Melanoma In Women." *Am J Epidemiol.* 134, no.5 (September 1991): 462–470.

9. F.C. Garland among others, "Occupational Sunlight Exposure and Melanoma in the U.S. Navy." *Arch Environ Health.* 45, no. 5 (1990): 261–7; Mark Elwood, "Melanoma and Sun Exposure." Vitasearch.com Expert Interview by Kirk Hamilton, 1997 (online July 2000). http://www.vitasearch.com/ CP/experts/melanoma2.htm (accessed Feb. 13, 2011); N. Hakansson among others, "Occupational Sunlight Exposure and Cancer Incidence Among Swedish Construction Workers." *Epidemiology.* 12, no. 5 (September 2001): 552–557; K.R. Cooke, D.C. Skegg, and J. Fraser, "Socio-econom-

ic Status, Indoor and Outdoor Work, and Malignant Melanoma." *Int J Cancer.* 34, no.1 (July 15, 1984): 57–62; M. Radespiel-Tröger among others, "Outdoor Work and Skin Cancer Incidence: a Registry-Based Study in Bavaria. *Int Arch Occup Environ Health.* 82, no. 3 (February 2009): 357–63. Epub 2008 Jul 23; K.R. Cooke, D.C. Skegg, and J. Fraser, "Socio-economic Status, Indoor and Outdoor Work, and Malignant Melanoma. *Int J Cancer.* 34, no. 1 (July 1984): 57–62; S. Gandini among others, "Meta-analysis of Risk Factors for Cutaneous Melanoma: II. Sun Exposure." *Eur J Cancer.* 41, no. 1 (January 2005): 45–60.

10. "Does Too Much Sun Cause Melanoma?" ScienceDaily. July 24, 2008. http://www.sciencedaily.com/releases/2008/07/080722192326.htm (accessed Mar 20, 2011); " 'Guardian Of The Genome' Protein Found To Underlie Skin Tanning." ScienceDaily. March 11, 2007. http://www.sciencedaily.com/releases/2007/03/070308122006.htm (accessed Mar 20, 2011); Moshe Oren and Jiri Bartek, "The Sunny Side of p53." Cell. 128, no. 5 (Mar. 9, 2007): 826-8; Rutao Cui among others, "Central Role of p53 in the Suntan Response and Pathologic Hyperpigmentation." Cell. 128, no 5 (Mar. 9, 2007): 853-864; M.A. Weinstock among others, "Melanoma and the Sun: the Effect of Swimsuits and a 'Healthy' Tan on the Risk of Nonfamilial Malignant Melanoma in Women." Am J Epidemiol. 134, no. 5 (Sept. 1, 1991): 462–70.

11. P. Autier, "Sunscreen Abuse for Intentional Sun Exposure." *Br J Dermatol.* 161, Supple 3 (November 2009): 40–5; J. Moan, A.C. Porojnicu, and A. Dahlback, "Ultraviolet Radiation and Malignant Melanoma." *Adv Exp Med Biol.* 624 (2008): 104-16; E.D. Gorham among others, "Do Sunscreens Increase Risk of Melanoma in Populations Residing at Higher Latitudes?" *Ann Epidemiol.* 17, no. 12 (December 2007): 956–63; C.F. Garland, F.C. Garland, and E.D. Gorham, "Epidemiologic Evidence for Different Roles of Ultraviolet A and B Radiation in Melanoma Mortality Rates." *Ann Epidemiol.* 13, no. 6 (July 2003): 395–404.

12. Edward Gorham, "Skin Cancer and Sunscreen Melanoma Cutaneous," Vitamin D Conference, December 2, 2008, U.C. San Diego, San Diego, California, www.grassrootshealth.org, http://www.ucsd.tv/search-details.aspx?showID=15770 (accessed Feb. 13, 2011).

13. Gregory Maltz, "Sunlight May Protect Against Cancers, Melanoma," *Family Practice News.* (February 1, 1996): 21. Vitasearch.com summary #24284A. http://www.vitasearch.com/get-clp-summary/15512 (accessed Feb. 13, 2011); J.F. Ashton and R.S. Laura, "Environmental Factors and the Etiology of Melanoma." *Cancer Causes Control.* 4, no. 1 (January 1993): 59–62; L. Bakos among others, "European Ancestry and Cutaneous Melanoma in Southern Brazil." *J Eur Acad Dermatol Venereol.* 23, no. 3 (March 2009): 304–7. Epub 2008 Dec 18; Erik L. Goldman, "Ten Common Myths Prevail About Melanoma." *Skin and Allergy News.* (July 1997): 14. Vitasearch.com summary #27927. http://www.vitasearch.com/get-clp-

summary/19069 (accessed Feb. 13, 2011); "Research Shows No Connection Between Tanning and Melanoma: Why This Is Misunderstood" (White Paper). Educational Institute for Indoor Tanning Salons, copyright 2006. International Smart Tan Network. http://www.electricbeachman-kato.com/images/Melanoma_Not_Related_to_Tanning.pdf (accessed Jan. 29, 2011); M.J. Eide and M.A.Weinstock, "Association of UV Index, Latitude, and Melanoma Incidence in Nonwhite Populations–US Surveillance, Epidemiology, and End Results (SEER) Program, 1992 to 2001. *Arch Dermatol.* 141, no 4 (April 2005): 477–81.

14. C.F. Garland, F.C. Garland, and E.D. Gorham, "Rising Trends in Melanoma. An Hypothesis Concerning Sunscreen Effectiveness." *Ann Epidemiol.* 1993 Jan;3(1):103–10.

15. William B Grant, *Cancer Survival, Ultraviolet-B Irradiation and Vitamin D.* Vitasearch.com Expert Speak interview by Kirk Hamilton, April 2006. http://www.vitasearch.com/CP/experts/WBGrantAT04-16-06.htm (accessed Feb. 13, 2011).

16. John Robbins, *Healthy at 100*. (New York: Ballantine Books, 2007); Dan Buettner, *The Blue Zones: Lessons for Living Longer From the People Who've Lived the Longest*. (Washington DC: National Geographic Society, 2008); Bradley J. Willcox, Craig Willcox, and Makoto Suzuki, *The Okinawa Program: How the World's Longest-Lived People Achieve Everlasting Health–And How You Can Too.* (New York: Three Rivers Press, 2001).

17. "Melanoma: What Are the Gaps in Our Knowledge?" *PLoS Med.* 5, no. 6 (June 2008): e122. http://www.ncbi.nlm.nih.gov/pmc/articles/PMC2408613/ (accessed Jan. 29, 2011); J.L. Rees among others, "The Melanoma Epidemic: Reality and Artefact." *BMJ.* 312, no.7024 (Jan. 20, 1996): 137–8; Sam Shuster, "Melanoma and Sun Exposure," *Lancet.* 346, no. 8984 (Nov. 4, 1995): 1224. Vitasearch.com summary #23504. http://www.vitasearch.com/get-clp-summary/16640 (accessed Feb. 13, 2011); J.S. MacNeil, "Sunlight and Vitamin D Controversy Heats Up: Endocrinologist Author Argues Exposure Promotes Vitamin D Production, Reduces Melanoma Risk." *Family Practice News.* (July 1, 2005): 28. Vitasearch.com summary #43379. http://www.vitasearch.com/get-clp-summary/34384 (accessed Feb. 13, 2011).

18. Yu-mei Chang and Jennifer H. Barrett, "Sun Exposure and Melanoma Risk at Different Latitudes: A Pooled Analysis of 5700 Cases and 7216 Controls." *Int J Epidemiol.* 38, no 3 (June 2009): 814–30. Epub 2009 Apr 8; E.A. Holly among others, "Cutaneous Melanoma in Women. I. Exposure to Sunlight, Ability to Tan, and Other Risk Factors Related to Ultraviolet Light. *Am J Epidemiol.* 141, no. 10 (May 1995): 923–33; L. Titus-Ernstoff among others, "A Relation Between Childhood Sun Exposure and Dysplastic Nevus Syndrome Among Patients with Nonfamilial Melanoma." *Epidemiology.* 2, no. 3 (May 1991): 210–4; J. Moan among others, "Ad-

dressing the Health Benefits and Risks, Involving Vitamin D or Skin Cancer, of Increased Sun Exposure. *Proc Natl Acad Sci USA*. 105, no. 2 (January 2008): 668–73. Epub 2008 Jan 7; P. Tuohimaa among others, "Does Solar Exposure, as Indicated by the Non-melanoma Skin Cancers, Protect from Solid Cancers: Vitamin D as a Possible Explanation." *Eur J Cancer*. 43, no. 11 (July 2007): 701–12. Epub 2007 May 30.

19. *Diabetes: Quick Diabetes Facts*. World Health Organization, Diabetes Programme. http://www.who.int/diabetes/en/index.html (accessed Feb. 13, 2011).

20. *Diabetes: How Can the Burden of Diabetes Be Reduced? Prevention*. World Health Organization, Media Centre, fact sheet no. 312, November 2009. http://www.who.int/mediacentre/factsheets/fs312/en/index.html (accessed Feb. 13, 2011).

21. *Basics About Diabetes: What are the Types of Diabetes?* Centers for Disease Control and Prevention, Diabetes Public Health Resource. http://www.cdc.gov/diabetes/consumer/learn.htm (accessed Feb. 13, 2011).

22. P.R. Njølstad among others, "Progress in Diabetes Genetics." *Tidsskr Nor Laegeforen*. 130, no 11 (June 3, 2010): 1145–9; J.K. Wolfordand B. Vozarova de Courten, "Genetic Basis of Type 2 Diabetes Mellitus: Implications for Therapy." *Treat Endocrinol*. 3, no. 4 (2004) 257–67; L. Qi, F.B. Hu, and G. Hu, "Genes, Environment, and Interactions in Prevention of Type 2 Diabetes: A Focus on Physical Activity and Lifestyle Changes." *Curr Mol Med*. 8, no. 6 (September 2008): 519–32.

23. D.O. Carpenter, "Environmental Contaminants as Risk Factors for Developing Diabetes." *Rev Environ Health*. 23, no. 1 (Jan.– Mar. 2008): 59–74; H.K. Son among others, "Strong Associations Between Low-dose Organochlorine Pesticides and Type 2 Diabetes in Korea." *Environ Int*. 36, no. 5 (July 2010): 410–4. Epub 2010 Apr 8.

24. N. Larsen among others, "Gut Microbiota in Human Adults with Type 2 Diabetes Differs from Non-diabetic Adults. *PLoS One*. 5, no. 2, (February 2010): e9085.

25. R.J. Barnard, T. Jung, and S.B. Inkeles, "Diet and Exercise in the Treatment of NIDDM. The Need For Early Emphasis. *Diabetes Care*. 17, no. 12 (December 1994): 1469–72; A.S. Nicholson and others, "Toward Improved Management of NIDDM: A Randomized, Controlled, Pilot Intervention Using a Low-fat, Vegetarian Diet." *Prev Med*. 29, no. 2 (August 1999): 87–91; D.J. Jenkins among others, "Type 2 Diabetes and the Vegetarian Diet." *Am J Clin Nutr*. 78., no. 3, 3 Suppl (September 2003): 610S–616S; N.D. Barnard among others, "A Low-fat Vegan Diet Improves Glycemic Control and Cardiovascular Risk Factors in a Randomized Clinical Trial in Individuals with Type 2 Diabetes." *Diabetes Care*. 29, no. 8 (August 2006): 1777–83; N.D. Barnard among others, "Vegetarian and Vegan Diets in

Type 2 Diabetes Management." *Nutr Rev.* 67, no. 5 (May 2009): 255–63; J.W. Anderson and K. Ward, "High-carbohydrate, High-fiber Diets for Insulin-treated Men with Diabetes Mellitus." *Am J Clin Nutr.* 32, no. 11 (November 1979): 2312–21; J.W. Anderson and P.B. Geil, "New Perspectives in Nutrition Management of Diabetes Mellitus." *Am J Med.* 85, no. 5A (November 1988): 159–65; C.C. Hamilton, P.B. Geil, and J.W. Anderson, "Management of Obesity in Diabetes Mellitus." *Diabetes Educ.* 18, no. 5 (Sept.–Oct. 1992): 407–10; J.W. Anderson, "Recent Advances in Carbohydrate Nutrition and Metabolism in Diabetes Mellitus." *J Am Coll Nutr.* 8, Suppl (1989): 61S–67S; J.W. Anderson, B.M. Smith, and P.B. Geil, "High-fiber Diet for Diabetes. Safe and Effective Treatment." *Postgrad Med.* 88, no. 2 (August 1990): 157–61, 164, 167–8; L.M. Goff among others, "Veganism and its Relationship with Insulin Resistance and Intramyocellular Lipid." *Eur J Clin Nutr.* 59, no. 2 (February 2005): 291–8; C.B. Trapp and N.D. Barnard, "Usefulness of Vegetarian and Vegan Diets for Treating Type 2 Diabetes." *Curr Diab Rep.* 10, no. 2 (April 2010): 152–8; H.I. Katcher among others, "A Worksite Vegan Nutrition Program is Well-accepted and Improves Health-related Quality of Life and Work Productivity." *Ann Nutr Metab.* 56, no. 4 (2010): 245–52. Epub 2010 Apr 14; S. Tonstad among others, "Type of Vegetarian Diet, Body Weight, and Prevalence of Type 2 Diabetes. *Diabetes Care.* 32, no. 5 (May 2009): 791–6. Epub 2009 Apr 7.

26. Kirk Hamilton, "Diabetes Reversal with the HCF Diet." Interview with James W. Anderson MD. *Staying Healthy Today Radio.* Prescription2000 website. April 30, 2009. http://www.prescription2000.com/Rx2000-Interviews-Podcast/diabetes-reversal-with-the-hcf-diet-an-interview-with-dr-james-anderson.html (accessed Feb. 13, 2011).

27. Kirk Hamilton, "Diabetes and Lipid Management Using the Dietary Portfolio, Nuts, Prebiotics and Soy." Interview with David JA Jenkins MD PhD DSc. *Staying Healthy Today Radio.* Prescription2000 website. March 11, 2010. http://www.prescription2000.com/Staying-Healthy-Today-Radio-Interviews/2010-03-11-david-jenkins-nuts-portfolio-prebiotic-soy.html (accessed Feb. 13, 2011); Kirk Hamilton, "Diabetes Reversal with the Portfolio Diet." Interview with David JA Jenkins MD PhD DSc. *Staying Healthy Today Radio.* Prescription2000 website. May 3, 2009. http://www.prescription2000.com/Rx2000-Interviews-Podcast/diabetes-reversal-with-the-portfolio-diet-an-interview-with-dr-david-jenkins.html (accessed Feb. 13, 2011).

28. Kirk Hamilton, "Diabetes Reversal Without Drugs." Interview with Neal Barnard MD. *Staying Healthy Today Radio.* Prescription2000 website. April 29, 2009. http://www.prescription2000.com/Rx2000-Interviews-Podcast/diabetes-reversal-without-drugs-an-interview-with-dr-neal-barnard.html (accessed Feb. 13, 2011).

29. Kirk Hamilton, "Diabetes Reversal with the *Eat For Health* Approach." Interview with Joel Fuhrman MD. *Staying Healthy Today Radio.* Prescrip-

tion2000 website. July 31, 2009. http://www.prescription2000.com/
Rx2000-Interviews-Podcast/2009-07-31-joel-fuhrman-md-diabetes.
html (accessed Feb. 13, 2011); Kirk Hamilton, "Chronic Disease Prevention and Reversal with the *Eat For Health* Program." Interview with Joel
Fuhrman MD. *Staying Healthy Today Radio.* Prescription2000 website.
July 31, 2009. http://www.prescription2000.com/Rx2000-Interviews-
Podcast/chronic-disease-reversal-dr-fuhrman.html (accessed Feb. 13,
2011). Kirk Hamilton, "Toxic Hunger, Weight Loss and the Benefits of
a High Micronutrient Dense Diet." Interview with Joel Fuhrman MD.
Staying Healthy Today Radio. Prescription2000 website. December 23,
2010. http://www.prescription2000.com/Staying-Healthy-Today-Radio-
Interviews/2010-12-23-joel-fuhrman-toxic-hunger-eat-to-live.html (accessed Feb. 13, 2011).

30. Kirk Hamilton, "Diabetes Reversal with the McDougall Program." Interview with John McDougall MD. *Staying Healthy Today Radio*, Prescrip-
tion2000 website. August 20, 2009. http://www.prescription2000.com/
Rx2000-Interviews-Podcast/2009-08-20-john-mcdougall-diabetes.html
(accessed Feb. 13, 2011).

31. *Diabetes Facts: Lack of Sufficient Diagnosis and Treatment.* World Diabetes
Foundation. http://www.worlddiabetesfoundation.org/composite-35.
htm (accessed Jan. 29, 2011); *Diabetes: What is Diabetes?* World Health
Organization, Media Centre, fact sheet no. 312, November 2009. http://
www.who.int/mediacentre/factsheets/fs312/en/index.html (accessed
Feb. 13, 2011).

32. C. Mathieu and K. Badenhoop, "Vitamin D and Type 1 Diabetes Mellitus:
State of the Art." *Trends Endocrinol Metab.* 16, no. 6 (August 2005): 261–
6; M.F. Holick, "High Prevalence of Vitamin D Inadequacy and Implica-
tions for Health." *Mayo Clin Proc.* 81, no. 3 (March 2006): 353–73; S.B.
Mohr among others, "Is There a Role of Vitamin D Deficiency in Type 1
Diabetes of Children?" *Am J Prev Med.* 39, no. 2 (August 2010): 189–90;
E. Hyppönen, "Vitamin D and Increasing Incidence of Type 1 Diabetes –
Evidence for an Association?" *Diabetes Obes Metab.* 12, no. 9 (September
2010): 737–43; Frank Garland, *Vitamin D and Diabetes – Can We Prevent it?* University of California Television, San Diego, February 5, 2009.
http://www.ucsd.tv/search-details.aspx?showID=15771 (accessed Feb.
13, 2011).

33. J. Lempainen among others, "Interplay between PTPN22 C1858T Poly-
morphism and Cow's Milk Formula Exposure in Type 1 Diabetes." *J Au-
toimmun.* 33, no. 2 (September 2009): 155–64. Epub 2009 May 26; K.
Luopajärvi among others, "Enhanced Levels of Cow's Milk Antibodies in
Infancy in Children who Develop Type 1 Diabetes Later in Childhood."
Pediatr Diabetes. 9, no. 5 (October 2008): 434–41. Epub 2008 May 21; E.
Skrodeniene among others, "Environmental Risk Factors in Prediction of
Childhood Prediabetes." *Medicina (Kaunas).* 44, no. 1 (2008): 56–63; G.

Soltesz, C.C. Patterson, and G. Dahlquist, EURODIAB Study Group, "World-wide Childhood Type 1 Diabetes Incidence – What can we Learn from Epidemiology?" *Pediatr Diabetes.* 8, Suppl 6 (October 2007): 6–14; O. Vaarala, "Is Type 1 Diabetes a Disease of the Gut Immune System Triggered by Cow's Milk Insulin?" *Adv Exp Med Biol.* 569 (2005): 151–6; J. Karjalainen among others, "A Bovine Albumin Peptide as a Possible Trigger of Insulin-dependent Diabetes Mellitus." *N Engl J Med.* 327, no. 5 (Jul. 30, 1992): 302–7; G. Frisk among others, "A Unifying Hypothesis on the Development of Type 1 Diabetes and Celiac Disease: Gluten Consumption May Be a Shared Causative Factor." *Med Hypotheses.* 70, no. 6 (2008):1207-9. Epub 2008 Feb 4; W. E. Barbeau among others, "Putting the Pieces of The Puzzle Together - A Series of Hypotheses on the Etiology and Pathogenesis of Type 1 Diabetes." *Med Hypotheses.* 68, no. 3 (2007):607-19. Epub 2006 Oct 11.

34. M. Serino among others, "Intestinal Microflora and Metabolic Diseases." *Diabetes Metab.* 35, no. 4 (September 2009): 262–72. Epub 2009 May 5; O. Vaarala, M.A. Atkinson, and J. Neu, "The 'Perfect Storm' for Type 1 Diabetes: the Complex Interplay Between Intestinal Microbiota, Gut Permeability, and Mucosal Immunity." *Diabetes.* 57, no. 10 (October 2008): 2555–62.

35. *Cardiovascular Ciseases (CVDs): What are the Risk Factors for Cardiovascular Disease?* World Health Organization, Media Centre, fact sheet no. 317, updated September 2009. http://www.who.int/mediacentre/factsheets/fs317/en/ (accessed Feb. 13, 2011).

36. *Cardiovascular Diseases (CVDs): How Can the Burden of Cardiovascular Diseases be Reduced?* World Health Organization, Media Centre, fact sheet no. 317, updated September 2009. http://www.who.int/mediacentre/factsheets/fs317/en/ (accessed Feb. 13, 2011).

37. *Cardiovascular Diseases (CVDs): How Can the Burden of Cardiovascular Diseases be Reduced?* World Health Organization, Media Centre, fact sheet no. 317, updated September 2009. http://www.who.int/mediacentre/factsheets/fs317/en/ (accessed Feb. 13, 2011).

38. *Cardiovascular Diseases (CVDs): How Can the Burden of Cardiovascular Diseases be Reduced?* World Health Organization, Media Centre, fact sheet no. 317, updated September 2009. http://www.who.int/mediacentre/factsheets/fs317/en/ (accessed Feb. 13, 2011).

39. *Cardiovascular Diseases (CVDs): How Can the Burden of Cardiovascular Diseases be Reduced?* World Health Organization, Media Centre, fact sheet no. 317, updated September 2009. http://www.who.int/mediacentre/factsheets/fs317/en/ (accessed Feb. 13, 2011).

40. *Step I, Step II and TLC Diets: What Does the TLC Diet Recommend?* American Heart Association. http://www.americanheart.org/presenter.jhtml?identifier=4764 (accessed Feb. 13, 2011).

41. *Nathan Pritikin: Founder*, The Pritikin Program. Pritikin Longevity Center and Spa. http://www.pritikin.com/index.php?option=com_content&view=article&id=61&Itemid=89 (accessed Jan. 29, 2011); L..M. Morrison, "Diet in Coronary Atherosclerosis." *J Am Med Assoc.* 173 (June 25, 1960): 884–8; L.M. Morrison, "A Nutritional Program for Prolongation of Life in Coronary Atherosclerosis." *J Am Med Assoc.* 159, no. 15 (December 1955): 1425–8; L.M. Morrison, "Diet and Atherosclerosis." *Ann Intern Med.* 37, no. 6 (December 1952): 1172–80; L.M. Morrison, "Reduction of Mortality Rate in Coronary Atherosclerosis by a Low Cholesterol-Low Fat Diet. *Am Heart J.* 42, no. 4 (October 1951): 538–45.

42. Dean Ornish among others, "Can Lifestyle Changes Reverse Coronary Heart Disease?" The Lifestyle Heart Trial. *Lancet.* 336, no. 8708 (July 21, 1990): 129–33.

43. Dean Ornish, *Dr. Dean Ornishs's Program For Reversing Heart Disease.* New York: Ballantine Books, 1996.

44. Richard M Fleming, *Stop Inflammation Now! A Step-by-Step Plan to Prevent, Treat, and Reverse Inflammation–The Leading Cause of Heart Disease and Related Conditions.* New York: G. P. Putnam's Sons, 2004.

45. Caldwell B. Esselstyn Jr., *Prevent and Reverse Heart Disease: The Revolutionary, Scientifically Proven, Nutrition-Based Cure.* New York: Avery – A Member of Penguin Group, 2008.

46. Rip Esselstyn. *The Engine 2 Diet: The Texas Firefighter's 28-Day Save-Your-Life Plan that Lowers Cholesterol and Burns Away the Pounds.* New York: Wellness Central, 2009.

47. T. Colin Campbell and Christine Cox, *The China Project: Revealing the Relationship Between Diet and Disease.* Trumansburg: The T. Colin Campbell Foundation, 2008:12–13.

48. Kirk Hamilton, "Heart Disease Risk, Cholesterol and Lipids in 2011: What Do We Really Know." Interview with William Castelli MD, *Staying Healthy Today Radio.* Prescription2000 website. February 18, 2011. http://www.prescription2000.com/Staying-Healthy-Today-Radio-Interviews/2011-02-18-william-castelli-heart-disease-lipids.html (accessed Feb. 21, 2011)

49. Kirk Hamilton, "Heart Disease Risk, Cholesterol and Lipids in 2011: What Do We Really Know." Interview with William Castelli MD, *Staying Healthy Today Radio.* Prescription2000 website. February 18, 2011. http://www.prescription2000.com/Staying-Healthy-Today-Radio-Interviews/2011-02-18-william-castelli-heart-disease-lipids.html (accessed Feb. 21, 2011)

50. Kirk Hamilton, "Heart Attack Proof ! How to Prevent and Reverse Heart Disease." Interview with Caldwell B. Esselstyn Jr MD. *Staying Healthy Today Radio*. Prescription2000 website. September 2, 2009. http://www.prescription2000.com/Rx2000-Interviews-Podcast/2009-09-02-caldwell-esselstyn-heart-attack.html (accessed Feb. 13, 2011).

51. Kirk Hamilton, "Heart Attack Proof ! How to Prevent and Reverse Heart Disease." Interview with Caldwell B. Esselstyn Jr MD. *Staying Healthy Today Radio*. Prescription2000 website. September 2, 2009. http://www.prescription2000.com/Rx2000-Interviews-Podcast/2009-09-02-caldwell-esselstyn-heart-attack.html (accessed Feb. 13, 2011).

52. Wolf Blitzer, *Clinton's Weight Loss Secret: Plants*. Interview with Bill Clinton. CNN website. September 22, 2010. http://www.cnn.com/video/#/video/us/2010/09/21/intv.clinton.blitzer.weight.loss.cnn?hpt=C2 (accessed Feb. 13, 2011).

53. Stephen T. Sinatra and James C. Roberts, *Reverse Heart Disease Now: Stop Deadly Cardiovascular Plaque Before It's Too Late.* (Hoboken, New Jersey: John Wiley & Sons Inc., 2007), 174–182; Kirk Hamilton, "Heart Disease Prevention and Reversal with the New Cardiology." Interview with Stephen Sinatra MD. *Staying Healthy Today Radio*. Prescription2000 website. June 3, 2010. http://www.prescription2000.com/Staying-Healthy-Today-Radio-Interviews/2010-06-03-stephen-sinatra-new-cardiology.html (accessed Feb. 13, 2011).

54. Kirk Hamilton, "Behavior Problems, Criminality and Food: The Undeniable Connection." Interview with Barbara Stitt PhD. *Staying Healthy Today Radio*. Prescription2000 website. May 30, 2009. http://www.prescription2000.com/Rx2000-Interviews-Podcast/dr-barbara-stitt-interview.html (accessed Feb. 13, 2011); Barbara Stitt, *Food and Behavior: A Natural Connection*. (Manitowoc, WI: Natural Press, 2004); Paul Stitt, *Beating the Food Giants*. (Manitowoc, WI: Natural Press, 1993).

55. Sanjay Gupta MD, Interview with Bill Clinton. Real Clear Politics website. March 11, 2009. http://www.realclearpolitics.com/articles/2009/03/interview_with_bill_clinton.html (accessed Feb. 13, 2011).

56. *President Obama's Fiscal 2010 Budget. Transforming and Modernizing America's Health Care System: Investing in Prevention and Wellness.* Office of Budget and Management. http://www.whitehouse.gov/omb/fy2010_key_healthcare/ (accessed Feb. 13, 2011).

57. *The Power of Prevention: Chronic Disease... the Public Health Challenge of the 21st Century.* Centers for Disease Control and Prevention. http://www.cdc.gov/chronicdisease/overview/index.htm http://www.cdc.gov/chronicdisease/pdf/2009-power-of-prevention.pdf (accessed Feb. 13, 2011).

58. *Ten Facts About Chronic Disease.* (1, 5, 10) World Health Organization. http://www.who.int/features/factfiles/chp/01_en.html (accessed Feb. 13, 2011).

59. Kirk Hamilton, "Chronic Disease Prevention and Reversal with a Plant-Based Diet and Lifestyle. Evidence From the "China Study" and a Life-time of Nutrition Research." Interview with T. Colin Campbell Ph.D. *Staying Healthy Today Radio.* Prescription2000 website. January 6, 2010. http://www.prescription2000.com/Staying-Healthy-Today-Radio-Interviews/2010-01-06-t-colin-campbell-phd-china-study.html (accessed Feb. 13, 2011).

Chapter 6
Expect Good Health!

1. J. Lazarou, B.H. Pomeranz, and P.N. Corey, "Incidence of Adverse Drug Reactions in Hospitalized Patients: A Meta-analysis of Prospective Studies. *JAMA.* 279, no. 15 (April 15, 1998): 1200–5.

Chapter 8
The Foundation for a *Staying Healthy* Diet

1. D.J. Jenkins among others, "Effect of a Diet High in Vegetables, Fruit, and Nuts on Serum Lipids." *Metabolism.* 46, no. 5 (May 1997): 530–7; Kirk Hamilton, "Lipids, Fruit, Nut and Vegetable Diet." Interview with David J.A. Jenkins MD PhD DSc. *Expert Speak Interviews.* Vitasearch website. July 2000. http://www.vitasearch.com/CP/experts/lipids3.htm (accessed Feb. 13, 2011).

2. *Paleolithic Diet* (definition), Wikipedia: The Free Encyclopedia. http://en.wikipedia.org/wiki/Paleolithic_diet (accessed Feb. 13, 2011).

3. Loren Cordain among others, "Plant-animal Subsistence Ratios and Macronutrient Energy Estimations in Worldwide Hunter-Gatherer Diets. *Am J Clin Nutr.* 71, no. 3 (March 2000):682-92; Kirk Hamilton, "The Paleolithic Diet–Pros and Cons in the 21st Century." Interview with Loren Cordain PhD. *Staying Healthy Today Radio.* Prescription2000 website. January 21, 2011. http://www.prescription2000.com/Staying-Healthy-Today-Radio-Interviews/2011-01-21-loren-cordain-paleo-diet.html (accessed Feb. 13, 2011).

4. Daphne Miller, *The Jungle Effect. A Doctor Discovers the Healthiest Diets from Around the World–Why They Work and How to Bring Them Home.* (New York: HarperCollins Publishers, 2008), 24.

5. Daphne Miller, *The Jungle Effect. A Doctor Discovers the Healthiest Diets from Around the World–Why They Work and How to Bring Them Home.* (New York: HarperCollins Publishers, 2008), 30-32, 36.

6. M. Nestle, "Animal v. Plant Foods in Human Diets and Health: Is the Historical Record Unequivocal? *Proc Nutr Soc.* 58, no. 2 (May 1999): 2118.

7. J.H. O'Keefe Jr. and L. Cordain, "Cardiovascular Disease Resulting From a Diet and Lifestyle at Odds With our Paleolithic Genome: How to Become a 21st-century Hunter-Gatherer. *Mayo Clin Proc.* 79, no. 1 (January 2004): 101–8.

8. D.C. Willcox among others, "The Okinawan Diet: Health Implications of a Low-calorie, Nutrient-dense, Antioxidant-rich Dietary Pattern Low in Glycemic Load." *J Am Coll Nutr.* 28 Suppl (August 2009): 500S–516S; B.J. Willcox among others, "Caloric Restriction, the Traditional Okinawan Diet, and Healthy Aging: The Diet of the World's Longest-lived People and its Potential Impact on Morbidity and Life Span." *Ann N Y Acad Sci.* 1114 (October 2007): 434–55; D.C. Willcox among others, "Aging Gracefully: A Retrospective Analysis of Functional Status in Okinawan Centenarians." *Am J Geriatr Psychiatry.* 15, no. 3 (March 2007): 252–6; D.C. Willcox among others, "The Cultural Context of 'Successful Aging' Among Older Women Weavers in a Northern Okinawan Village: The Role of Productive Activity." *J Cross Cult Gerontol.* 22, no. 2 (June 2007): 137-65; A.M. Bernstein among others, "First Autopsy Study of an Okinawan Centenarian: Absence of Many Age-related Diseases." *J Gerontol A Biol Sci Med Sci.* 59, no. 11 (November 2004): 1195–9; M. Akisaka, Y. Tanaka, and M. Suzuki, "Longitudinal and Comprehensive Follow-up Study of the Oldest Man in Japan." *Nippon Ronen Igakkai Zasshi.* 34, no. 4 (April 1997): 312–23; M. Akisaka among others, "Energy and Nutrient Intakes of Okinawan Centenarians." *J Nutr Sci Vitaminol* (Tokyo). 42, no. 3 (June 1996): 241–8; M. Suzuki among others, "Chronological Study Concerning ADL Among Okinawan Centenarians." *Nippon Ronen Igakkai Zasshi.* 32, no 6 (June 1995): 416-23.

9. Sanjay Gupta, "Western Diet: A Killer in Okinawa. Part II." Vita+Signs, CNN You Tube. http://www.youtube.com/watch?v=8teAABsnTmM&feature= related (accessed Feb. 13, 2011).

10. Bradley J. Willcox, D. Craig Willcox, and Makoto Suzuki, *The Okinawa Diet Plan: the Only Diet with 100 Years of Living Proof* (New York: Three Rivers Press, 2004), 46, 57.

11. Dan Buettner, *The Blue Zone: Lessons for Living Longer from the People Who've Lived the Longest.* (Washington DC: National Geographic Society, 2008), 48-49, 59.

12. Gerard Anderson, "Chronic Conditions: Making the Case for Ongoing Care." Baltimore, MD: John Hopkins University; November, 2007: 16, 22,

25. http://www.fightchronicdisease.org/news/pfcd/documents/Chron-icCareChartbook_FINAL.pdf (accessed Feb. 15, 2011) ; *The Power of Prevention Chronic Disease ... The Public Health Challenge of the 21st Century, 2009*, Department of Health and Human Services – USA, National Center For Chronic Disease Prevention and Healthy Promotion, Centers for Disease Control: 1. http://www.cdc.gov/chronicdisease/pdf/2009-Power-of-Prevention.pdf (accessed Feb. 12, 2011).

13. Loren Cordain, "Cereal Grains: Humanity's Double-Edge Sword." *World Rev Nutr Diet.* 84 (1999):23-24; Kirk Hamilton, "The Paleolithic Diet – Pros and Cons in the 21st Century." Interview with Loren Cordain PhD. *Staying Healthy Today Radio*. Prescription2000 website. January 21, 2011. http://www.prescription2000.com/Staying-Healthy-Today-Radio Interviews/2011-01-21-loren-cordain-paleo-diet.html; http://www.prescription2000.com/images/stories/transcripts/2011-01-21-loren-cordain-paleo-diet-transcript.pdf , pages 3, 8 (accessed Feb. 13, 2011).

14. D.J. Jenkins among others, "A Dietary Portfolio Approach to Cholesterol Reduction: Combined Effects of Plant Sterols, Vegetable Proteins, and Viscous Fibers in Hypercholesterolemia." *Metabolism.* 51, no. 12 (December 2002): 1596–604; D.J. Jenkins among others, "Effects of a Dietary Portfolio of Cholesterol-Lowering Foods vs. Lovastatin on Serum Lipids and C-reactive Protein." *JAMA.* 290, no. 4 (July 23, 2003): 502–10; D.J. Jenkins among others, "Type 2 Diabetes and the Vegetarian Diet." *Am J Clin Nutr.* 78, 3 Suppl (September 2003): 610S–616S.

15. Kirk Hamilton, "Diabetes Reversal with the Portfolio Diet." Interview with David J.A. Jenkins MD PhD DSc. *Staying Healthy Today Radio*, Prescription2000 website. May 3, 2009, 8–9 (pdf transcript). http://www.prescription2000.com/images/stories/transcripts/2009-05-03_DJAJenkins_transcript.pdf ; http://www.prescription2000.com/Rx2000-Interviews-Podcast/diabetes-reversal-with-the-portfolio-diet-an-interview-with-dr-david-jenkins.html (accessed Feb. 13, 2011).

16. *Country Comparison: Population*. The World Factbook. Central Intelligence Agency website. https://www.cia.gov/library/publications/the-world-factbook/geos/ch.html (accessed Feb. 20, 2011).

17. United States Department of Agriculture (USDA), National Agricultural Statistics Service (NASS). *Poultry Slaughter 2009 Summary.* February 2010, Pou 2-1 (10), page 2. http://usda.mannlib.cornell.edu/usda/current/PoulSlauSu/PoulSlauSu-02-25-2010.pdf (accessed Jan. 29, 2011).; United States Department of Agriculture (USDA), National Agricultural Statistics Service (NASS). *Livestock Slaughter 2009 Summary.* April 2010, Mt An 1-2 -1 (10), page 1. http://usda.mannlib.cornell.edu/usda/current/LiveSlauSu/LiveSlauSu-04-29-2010.pdf (accessed Feb. 13, 2011).

18. James H. O'Keefe Jr. and Loren Cordain, "Cardiovascular Disease Resulting From a Diet and Lifestyle at Odds with Our Paleolithic Genome: How to

Become a 21st-Century Hunter-Gatherer." *Mayo Clin Proc.* 79 (2004): 105. http://www.mayoclinicproceedings.com/content/79/1/101.full.pdf (accessed Feb. 13, 2011).

19. Joel Fuhrman, *Eat To Live: The Revolutionary Formula for Fast and Sustained Weight Loss.* Revised Edition. (New York: Little, Brown and Company, 2011), 71.

20. Compiled with the assistance of the *VegNews* magazine staff. Compliments of Colleen Holland, associate publisher. *VegNews*, 3620 Wawona Street, San Francisco, CA 94116, 415-665-6397 / 415-665-6398 (FAX), vegnews.com.

21. Tony Gonzalez with Mitzi Dulan, *The All-Pro Diet: Lose Fat, Build Muscle, and Live Like a Champion.* (New York: Rodale Books, 2009), 40.

22. Tony Gonzalez with Mitzi Dulan, *The All-Pro Diet: Lose Fat, Build Muscle, and Live Like a Champion.* (New York: Rodale Books, 2009).

Chapter 9
Double Trouble? Dairy and Grains

1. A.J. Lanou, "Should Dairy be Recommended as Part of a Healthy Vegetarian Diet? Counterpoint." *Am J Clin Nutr.* 89, no. 5 (May 2009): 1638S–39S. Epub 2009 Mar 25; D. Feskanich among others, "Milk, Dietary Calcium, and Bone Fractures In Women: A 12-Year Prospective Study." *Am J Public Health.* 87, no. 6 (June 1997) :992-7; K. Michaëlsson among others, "Dietary Calcium and Vitamin D Intake in Relation to Osteoporotic Fracture Risk." *Bone.* 32, no. 6 (June 2003) :694-703; H.A Bischoff-Ferrari among others, "Calcium Intake and Hip Fracture Risk in Men and Women: A Meta-Analysis of Prospective Cohort Studies and Randomized Controlled Trials." *Am J Clin Nutr.* 86, no. 6 (December 2007) :1780-90; J. A. Kanis among others, "A Meta-Analysis of Milk Intake and Fracture Risk: Low Utility for Case Finding." *Osteoporos Int.* 16, no. 7 (July 2005): 799-804. Epub 2004 Oct 21.

2. A.J. Lanou, "Should Dairy be Recommended as Part of a Healthy Vegetarian Diet? Counterpoint." *Am J Clin Nutr.* 89, no. 5 (May 2009): 1638S. Epub 2009 Mar 25.

3. A.J. Lanou, "Should Dairy be Recommended as Part of a Healthy Vegetarian Diet? Counterpoint." *Am J Clin Nutr.* 89, no. 5 (May 2009): 1639S. Epub 2009 Mar 25; B.J. Abelow among others, "Cross-Cultural Association Between Dietary Animal Protein and Hip Fracture: A Hypothesis." *Calcif Tissue Int.* 50, no. 1 (January 1992): 14-8; N.A. Breslau among others, "Relationship of Animal Protein-Rich Diet to Kidney Stone Formation and Calcium Metabolism." *J Clin Endocrinol Metab.* 66, no. 1 (January 1988):

140-6; U.S. Barzel among others, "Excess Dietary Protein Can Adversely Affect Bone." *J Nutr.* 128, no. 6 (June 1998): 1051-3; L. Frassetto among others, "Diet, Evolution and Aging-The Pathophysiologic Effects of The Post-Agricultural Inversion of the Potassium-to-Sodium and Base-to-Chloride Ratios in the Human Diet." *Eur J Nutr.* 40, no. 5 (October 2001): 200-13.

4. Kirk Hamilton, "The Paleolithic Diet – Pros and Cons in the 21st Century." Interview with Loren Cordain PhD. *Staying Healthy Today Radio.* Prescription2000 website. January 21, 2011. http://www.prescription2000.com/Staying-Healthy-Today-Radio-Interviews/2011-01-21-loren-cordain-paleo-diet.html (accessed Feb. 13, 2011); http://www.prescription2000.com/images/stories/transcripts/2011-01-21-loren-cordain-paleo-diet-transcript.pdf, page 6. (accessed Feb. 20, 2011)

5. Dan Buettner, *The Blue Zone: Lessons for Living Longer from the People Who've Lived the Longest.* (Washington DC: National Geographic Society, 2008), 59.

6. Dan Buettner, *The Blue Zone: Lessons for Living Longer from the People Who've Lived the Longest.* (Washington DC: National Geographic Society, 2008), 239–243.

7. Amy Joy Lanou and Michael Castelman, *Building Better Bone Vitality: A Revolutionary Diet Plan to Prevent Bone Loss and Reverse Osteoporosis.* (New York: McGraw-Hill Companies, Inc, 2009), 3–8 and 209–222 (Appendix A).

8. Amy Joy Lanou and Michael Castelman, Building Better Bone Vitality: A Revolutionary Diet Plan to Prevent Bone Loss and Reverse Osteoporosis. (New York: McGraw-Hill Companies, Inc, 2009), 121–124.

9. A.J. Lanou, "Should Dairy be Recommended as Part of a Healthy Vegetarian Diet? Counterpoint." *Am J Clin Nutr.* 89, vol. 5 (May 2009): 1640S (Table:2). Epub 2009 Mar 25; D. Ganmaa and A. Sato, "The Possible Role of Female Sex Hormones in Milk From Pregnant Cows in the Development of Breast, Ovarian and Corpus Uteri Cancers." *Med Hypotheses.* 65, no. 6 (2005): 1028–37. Epub 2005 Aug 24; S.C. Larsson, N. Orsini, and A. Wolk, "Milk, Milk Products and Lactose Intake and Ovarian Cancer Risk: A Meta-analysis of Epidemiological Studies." *Int J Cancer.* 118, no. 2 (Jan. 15, 2006): 431–41; L.Q. Qin among others, "Milk/Dairy Products Consumption, Galactose Metabolism and Ovarian Cancer: Meta-analysis of Epidemiological Studies." *Eur J Cancer Prev.* 14, no. 1 (February 2005): 13–9; X.M. Li, D. Ganmaa, and A. Sato, "The Experience of Japan as a Clue to the Etiology of Breast and Ovarian Cancers: Relationship Between Death from both Malignancies and Dietary Practices." *Med Hypotheses.* 60, no. 2 (February 2003): 268–75; J.M. Genkinger among others, "Dairy Products and Ovarian Cancer: A Pooled Analysis of 12 Cohort Studies." *Cancer Epidemiol Biomarkers Prev.* 15 (2006): 364–72; World Cancer Research

Fund, American Institute for Cancer Research. *Food, Nutrition, Physical Activity, and the Prevention of Cancer: A Global Perspective.* Washington DC: AICR, 2007; E. Giovannucci among others, "Calcium and Fructose Intake in Relation to Risk of Prostate Cancer. *Cancer Res.* 58 (1998): 442–447; E. Giovannucci among others, "Risk Factors for Prostate Cancer Incidence and Progression" in the Health Professionals Follow-up Study. *International Journal of Cancer.* 121 (2007): 1571–78.

10. Praveen K. Roy among others., *Lactose Intolerance*, eMedicine from Web MD, August 12, 2008. http://emedicine.medscape.com/article/187249-overview (accessed Jan. 29, 2011).

11. *Foods Highest in Saturated Fat (based on levels per 200-calorie serving) in DairyandEggProducts,*SelfNutritionData:KnowWhatYouEat,NutritionData.com. http://nutritiondata.self.com/foods-00101600000000000000.html?maxCount=113 (accessed Feb. 13, 2011).

12. *How Much Do I Need? Vitamin D.* Harvard School of Public Health. http://www.hsph.harvard.edu/nutritionsource/what-should-you-eat/vitamin-d/index.html (accessed Sept. 25, 2010); *Vitamin D and Your Health. How Much Vitamin D Should I Take: What We Recommend.* Vitamin D Council. http://www.vitamindcouncil.org/health/deficiency/am-i-vitamin-d-deficient.shtml (accessed Feb. 13, 2011).

13. K. Luopajärvi among others, "Enhanced Levels of Cow's Milk Antibodies in Infancy in Children who Develop Type 1 Diabetes Later in Childhood." *Pediatr Diabetes.* 9, no. 5 (October 2008): 434–41. Epub 2008 May 21; M.F. Goldfarb, "Relation of Time of Introduction of Cow Milk Protein to an Infant and Risk of Type 1 Diabetes Mellitus." *J Proteome Res.* 7, no. 5 (May 2008): 2165–7. Epub 2008 Apr 15; E. Skrodeniene among others, "Environmental Risk Factors in Prediction of Childhood Prediabetes." *Medicina (Kaunas).* 44, no. 1 (2008): 56–63; B. Banwell among others, Wadsworth Pediatric Multiple Sclerosis Study Group. "Abnormal T-cell Reactivities in Childhood Inflammatory Demyelinating Disease and Type 1 Diabetes." *Ann Neurol.* 63, no. 1 (January 2008): 98–111; K. Dahl-Jørgensen, G. Joner, and K.F. Hanssen, "Relationship Between Cows' Milk Consumption and Incidence of IDDM in Childhood." *Diabetes Care.* 14, no. 11 (November 1991): 1081–3.

14. *Understanding the Problems with Dairy Products. Understanding the Problems with Dairy Products: 8. Health Concerns of Infants and Children.* NutritionMD. http://www.nutritionmd.org/nutrition_tips/nutrition_tips_understand_foods/dairy.html (accessed Feb. 13, 2011).

15. *Cow's milk for infants and children: Recommendations.* MedlinePlus. http://www.nlm.nih.gov/medlineplus/ency/article/002448.htm (accessed Feb. 13, 2011).

16. G. Iacono among others, "Intolerance of Cow's Milk and Chronic Consti-
    pation in Children." *N Engl J Med.* 339, (1998): 110–4; M.A. El-Hodhod
    among others, "Cow's Milk Allergy Related Pediatric Constipation: Ap-
    propriate Time of Milk Tolerance." *Pediatr Allergy Immunol.* 21, no. 2, Pt 2
    (March 2010): e407–12. Epub 2009 Jun 25; K.F. Michaelsen among oth-
    ers, "Whole Cow's Milk: Why, What and When?" *Nestle Nutr Workshop
    Ser Pediatr Program.* 60 (2007): 201–16; discussion 216–9; E.E. Ziegler,
    "Adverse Effects of Cow's Milk in Infants." *Nestle Nutr Workshop Ser Pedi-
    atr Program.* 60 (2007): 185–96; discussion 196–9.

17. Richard Hamilton, "Agriculture's Sustainable Future: Breeding Bet-
    ter Crops Modern Technologies Can Increase Crop Yields and Reduce
    Agriculture's Environmental Impact." *Scientific American,* June 2009
    (on line July 15, 2009). http://www.scientificamerican.com/article.
    cfm?id=agricultures-sustainable-future (accessed Feb. 13, 2011).

18. John Robbins, *Healthy at 100.* (New York: Ballantine Books, 2007); Dan
    Buettner, *The Blue Zones: Lessons for Living Longer From the People
    Who've Lived the Longest.* (Washington DC: National Geographic Society,
    2008); Bradley J. Willcox, D. Craig Willcox, and Makoto Suzuki, *The Oki-
    nawa Program: How the World's Longest-Lived People Achieve Everlasting
    Health–And How You Can Too.* (New York: Three Rivers Press, 2001).

19. Susan Mattingly, *Whole Grains. California Food Guide: Fulfilling the Di-
    etary Guidelines for Americans.* Chapter 3. August 25, 2006, 1–2. http://
    www.dhcs.ca.gov/dataandstats/reports/documents/californiafood-
    guide /3wholegrain.pdf (accessed Jan. 29, 2011); Jean Buzby, Hodan
    Farah, and Gary Vocke, "Will 2005 Be the Year of the Whole Grain?" *Am-
    berWaves.* June 2005. http://www.ers.usda.gov/AmberWaves/June05/
    Features/Will2005WholeGrain.htm (accessed Feb. 13, 2011).

20. Susan Mattingly, *Whole Grains. California Food Guide: Fulfilling the Dietary
    Guidelines for Americans.* Chapter 3. August 25, 2006, 5. http://www.
    dhcs.ca.gov/dataandstats/reports/documents/californiafoodguide/
    3wholegrain.pdf (accessed Feb. 13, 2011).

21. Jean Buzby, Hodan Farah, and Gary Vocke, "Will 2005 Be the Year of the
    Whole Grain?" *AmberWaves,* June 2005. http://www.ers.usda.gov/Am-
    berWaves/June05/Features/Will2005WholeGrain.htm (accessed Feb.
    13, 2011).

22. Jean Buzby, Hodan Farah, and Gary Vocke, "Will 2005 Be the Year of the
    Whole Grain?" *AmberWaves,* June 2005. http://www.ers.usda.gov/Am-
    berWaves/June05/Features/Will2005WholeGrain.htm (accessed Feb.
    13, 2011).

23. Lisa Mancino and Jean Buzby, *Americans' Whole-Grain Consumption Be-
    low Guidelines.* http://www.ers.usda.gov/Amberwaves/April05/pdf/
    april05_findings_wholegrainconsumption.pdf (accessed Feb. 13, 2011).

24. Loren Cordain, "Cereal Grains: Humanity's Double-Edge Sword." *World Rev Nutr Diet*. 84 (1999):19-73;   Kirk Hamilton, "The Paleolithic Diet – Pros and Cons in the 21st Century." Interview with Loren Cordain PhD. *Staying Healthy Today Radio*. Prescription2000 website. January 21, 2011. http://www.prescription2000.com/Staying-Healthy-Today-Radio-Interviews/2011-01-21-loren-cordain-paleo-diet.html (accessed Feb. 13, 2011).

Chapter 10
The Big Three: Alcohol, Caffeine, and Sugar

1. *Alcoholic Beverages, Key Recommendations*, Dietary Guidelines for Americans 2005. Chapter 9. United States Department of Agriculture. Updated July 9, 2008. http://www.health.gov/DIETARYGUIDELINES/dga2005/document/html/chapter9.htm (accessed Feb. 13, 2011).

2. Kirk Hamilton, "Caffeine Withdrawal and Cardiovascular Risk." Interview with Jack E. James, *The Experts Speak*. Vitasearch website. http://www.vitasearch.com/CP/experts/caffeine.htm (accessed Feb. 13, 2011).

3. Kirk Hamilton, "Depression, Caffeine and Sugar." Interview with Larry Christensen, *The Experts Speak*. Vitasearch website. http://www.vitasearch.com/CP/experts/depression6.htm (accessed Feb. 13, 2010).

4. Larry Dolce, "How Caffeine Can Affect Your Health." Ezine Articles website. http://ezinearticles.com/?How-Caffeine-Can-Affect-Your-Health&id=101557 (accessed Feb. 13, 2011).

5. *Thrifty Gene Hypothesis*. Wikipedia the Free Encyclopedia. Wikipedia website. Modified on 1 August 2010 at 23:09. http://en.wikipedia.org/wiki/Thrifty_gene_hypothesis (accessed Feb. 13, 2011); James V. Neel, "Diabetes Mellitus: A 'Thrifty' Genotype Rendered Detrimental by 'Progress'?" PubMed Central website. http://www.ncbi.nlm.nih.gov/pmc/articles/PMC1932342/pdf/ajhg00558-0047.pdf (accessed Feb. 13, 2011).

6. *High Fructose Corn Syrup*. Wikipedia the Free Encyclopedia. Wikipedia website. Modified on 7 February 2011 at 10:29. en.wikipedia.org/wiki/High_fructose_corn_syrup (accessed Feb. 13, 2011);   "What is HFCS (High Fructose Corn Syrup)?" SweetSuprise.com Corn Refiners Association (CRA) website. http://sweetsurprise.com/learning-center/what-is-hfcs?utm_source=google&utm_medium=cpc&utm_term=fructose%20corn%20sugar&utm_campaign=cornsugar_cornsugar&gclid=CJ-0uLiEpqQCFQ5biAodQCef4g (accessed Feb. 13, 2011).

7. J. Pihlajamäki among others, "Insulin Resistance is Associated with Increased Cholesterol Synthesis and Decreased Cholesterol Absorption in

Normoglycemic Men." *J Lipid Res*. 45, no. 3 (March 2004): 507–12. Epub 2003 Dec 1.

8. Elaine Gloria Gottschall, *Breaking the Vicious Cycle: Intestinal Health Through Diet*. Thirteenth Edition. (Baltimore, Ontario, Canada: Kirkton Press Ltd, 2010).

9. *Brain Energy Demand*. The Franklin Institute: Resources for Science Learning. http://www.fi.edu/learn/brain/carbs.html#brainenergy (accessed Feb. 13, 2011).

10. *Brain Power – The Energy of Thought and Memory*. The Franklin Institute: Resources for Science Learning. http://www.fi.edu/learn/brain/carbs. html#brainenergy (accessed Feb. 13, 2011).

11. *Too Much Blood Sugar –Too Little Brain Sugar*. The Franklin Institute: Resources for Science Learning. http://www.fi.edu/learn/brain/carbs. html#brainenergy (accessed Feb. 13, 2011).

Chapter 12
"Allergic Load" and Detoxification

1. C.A. Clemetson, "Histamine and Ascorbic Acid in Human Blood." *J Nutr*. 110, no. 4 (April 1980) : 662–8; P. Patak, H.S. Willenberg, and S. R. Bornstein, "Vitamin C is an Important Cofactor for Both Adrenal Cortex and Adrenal Medulla." *Endocr Res*. 30, no. 4 (November 2004): 871–5.

2. G.I. Betsi, E. Papadavid, and M.E. Falagas, "Probiotics for the Treatment or Prevention of Atopic Dermatitis: A Review of the Evidence from Randomized Controlled Trials." *Am J Clin Dermatol*. 9, no. 2 (2008): 93–103; B.R. Goldin and S.L. Gorbach, "Clinical Indications for Probiotics: An Overview." *Clin Infect Dis*. 46, Suppl 2 (Feb. 1, 2008): S96–100; discussion S144–51.

3. L.E. Morrow, "Probiotics in the Intensive Care Unit." *Curr Opin Crit Care*. 15, no. 2 (April 2009): 144–8; K. Madsen, "Probiotics in Critically Ill Patients." *J Clin Gastroenterol*. 42, Suppl 3 Pt 1 (September 2008): S116–8.

4. Report of a Joint FAO/WHO Expert Consultation on Evaluation of Health and Nutritional Properties of Probiotics in Food Including Powder Milk with Live Lactic Acid Bacteria. *Health and Nutritional Properties of Probiotics in Food including Powder Milk with Live Lactic Acid Bacteria Report*. Amerian Córdoba Park Hotel, Córdoba, Argentina, October 1-4, 2001: 5. http://www.who.int/foodsafety/publications/fs_management/en/probiotics.pdf (accessed Feb. 13, 2011).

5. M. Heyman, "Gut Barrier Dysfunction in Food Allergy." *Eur J Gastroenterol Hepatol*. 2005 Dec;17(12):1279–85.

6. W.A. Walker, "Antigen Absorption from the Small Intestine and Gastrointestinal Disease." *Pediatr Clin North Am.* 22, no. 4 (November 1975): 731–46.

7. H. Needleman, "Low Level Lead Exposure: History and Discovery." *Ann Epidemiol.* 19, no. 4 (April 2009): 235–8; H. Needleman, "Standing up to the Lead Industry: An Interview with Herbert Needleman." Interview by David Rosner and Gerald Markowitz. *Public Health Rep.* 120, no. 3 (May-Jun 2005): 330-7. PDF of entire interview available at: http://www.ncbi.nlm.nih.gov/pmc/articles/PMC1497712/pdf/16134577.pdf   (accessed Feb. 13, 2011).

8. Kirk Hamilton, "Chronic Disease Reversal Using Medically Supervised Fasting and Healthy Living With Dietary Avoidance of the "Pleasure Trap" Foods." Interview with Alan Goldhamer, D.C., *Staying Healthy Today Radio.* Prescription2000 website. April 28, 2010. http://www.prescription2000.com/Staying-Healthy-Today-Radio-Interviews/2010-04-28-alan-goldhamer-fasting.html (accessed Feb. 13, 2011).

Chapter 13
The TRIAD Diet Program

1. Joel Fuhrman, *Eat To Live: The Revolutionary Formula for Fast and Sustained Weight Loss.* Revised Edition. (New York: Little, Brown and Company, 2011), 7.

2. Joel Fuhrman, *Eat For Health, Book One–The Mind Makeover.* First Edition. (Flemington, New Jersey: Gift of Health Press, 2008), 49–55; Joel Fuhrman, *Eat For Health, Book Two–The Body Makeover.* First Edition. (Flemington, New Jersey: Gift of Health Press, 2008), 9.

3. Bradley J. Willcox, D. Craig Willcox, and Makoto Suzuki, *The Okinawa Diet Plan: the Only Diet with 100 Years of Living Proof* (New York: Three Rivers Press, 2004), 49–51; Bradley J. Willcox, D. Craig Willcox, and Makoto Suzuki, *The Okinawa Diet Plan: The Only Diet with 100 years of Living Proof* (New York: Three Rivers Press, 2004), 53.

4. Bradley J. Willcox, D. Craig Willcox, and Makoto Suzuki, *The Okinawa Diet Plan: The Only Diet with 100 years of Living Proof* (New York: Three Rivers Press, 2004), 58–60.

5. Bradley J. Willcox, D. Craig Willcox, and Makoto Suzuki, *The Okinawa Diet Plan: The Only Diet with 100 Years of Living Proof* (New York: Three Rivers Press, 2004), 56.

6. Barbara Rolls, *The Volumetrics Eating Plan: Techniques and Recipies for Feeling Full on Fewer Calories* (New York: Harper, 2007).

7. Joel Fuhrman, *Eat To Live: The Revolutionary Formula for Fast and Sustained Weight Loss*. Revised Edition. (New York: Little, Brown and Company, 2011), 116.

8. Kirk Hamilton, *Chronic Disease Prevention and Reversal With The "Eat For Health" Program*. Interview with Joel Fuhrman MD, *Staying Healthy Today Radio*. Prescription2000.com. July 31, 2009. (pdf transcript): 9. http://www.prescription2000.com/images/stories/transcripts/2009-07-31-joel-fuhrman-chronic-disease-transcripts.pdf; audio interview http://www.prescription2000.com/Rx2000-Interviews-Podcast/chronic-disease-reversal-dr-fuhrman.html (accessed Feb. 13, 2011).

9. F.B. Fu among others, "Frequent Nut Consumption and Risk of Coronary Heart Disease in Women: Prospective Cohort Study. *BMJ*. 317, no. 7169 (November 1998): 1341–5.

10. C.M. Albert among others, "Nut Consumption and Decreased Risk of Sudden Cardiac Death in the Physicians' Health Study. *Arch Intern Med*. 162, no. 12 (June 2002): 1382–7.

11. P.M. Kris-Etherton among others, "The Role of Tree Nuts and Peanuts in the Prevention of Coronary Heart Disease: Multiple Potential Mechanisms." *J Nutr*. 138, no. 9 (September 2008): 1746S-1751S.

12. J. Sabaté and Y. Ang, "Nuts and Health Outcomes: New Epidemiologic Evidence." *Am J Clin Nutr*. 89, no. 5 (May 2009): 1643S–1648S. Epub 2009 Mar 25.

13. Panel on Dietary Reference Intakes for Electrolytes and Water, Standing Committee on the Scientific Evaluation of Dietary Reference Intakes, Food and Nutrition Board, Institute Of Medicine Of The National Academies. *Dietary Reference Intakes: Water, Potassium, Sodium, Chloride, and Sulfate. Chapter 4. Water*. (Washington, DC: The National Academies Press, 2005), 73. http://books.nap.edu/openbook.php?record_id=10925&page=73 (accessed Feb. 13, 2011).

14. L. Ryan and S. Petit, "Addition of Whole, Semi-skimmed, and Skimmed Bovine Milk Reduces the Total Antioxidant Capacity of Black Tea." *Nutr Res*. 30, no. 1 (January 2010): 14–20.

15. J.V. Higdon and B. Frei, "Tea Catechins and Polyphenols: Health Effects, Metabolism, and Antioxidant Functions." *Crit Rev Food Sci Nutr*. 43, no. 1 (2003): 89–143.

16. H. Sung among others, "In Vivo Antioxidant Effect of Green Tea." *Eur J Clin Nutr*. 54, no. (July 2000): 527–9.

17. J. Lempainen among others, "Interplay between PTPN22 C1858T Polymorphism and Cow's Milk Formula Exposure in Type 1 Diabetes." *J Autoimmun*. 33, no. 2 (September 2009): 155–64. Epub 2009 May 26; K. Luopajärvi among others, "Enhanced Levels of Cow's Milk Antibodies in

Infancy in Children who Develop Type 1 Diabetes Later in Childhood." *Pediatr Diabetes.* 9, no. 5 (October 2008): 434–41. Epub 2008 May 21; E. Skrodeniene among others, "Environmental Risk Factors in Prediction of Childhood Prediabetes." *Medicina (Kaunas).* 44, no. 1 (2008): 56–63; G. Soltesz, C.C. Patterson, and G. Dahlquist, EURODIAB Study Group, "World-wide Childhood Type 1 Diabetes Incidence – What can we Learn from Epidemiology?" *Pediatr Diabetes.* 8, Suppl 6 (October 2007): 6–14; O. Vaarala, "Is Type 1 Diabetes a Disease of the Gut Immune System Triggered by Cow's Milk Insulin?" *Adv Exp Med Biol.* 569 (2005): 151–6; J. Karjalainen among others, "A Bovine Albumin Peptide as a Possible Trigger of Insulin-dependent Diabetes Mellitus." *N Engl J Med.* 327, no. 5 (Jul. 30, 1992): 302–7; G. Frisk and others, "A Unifying Hypothesis on the Development of Type 1 Diabetes and Celiac Disease: Gluten Consumption May Be a Shared Causative Factor." *Med Hypotheses.* 70, no. 6 (2008):1207-9. Epub 2008 Feb 4; W. E. Barbeau among others, "Putting the Pieces of The Puzzle Together - A Series of Hypotheses on the Etiology and Pathogenesis of Type 1 Diabetes." *Med Hypotheses.* 68, no. 3 (2007):607-19. Epub 2006 Oct 11.

18. Joel Fuhrman among others, "Changing Perceptions of Hunger on a High Nutrient Density Diet. *Nutrition Journal.* 9 (Nov. 7, 2010): 51.

Chapter 14
The TRIAD Exercise Program

1. The Nielsen Company, "What Consumers Watch: Americans Spend More Time with Video Than Ever Consumers devote 3.5 hours a month to using TV and the Internet simultaneously." *Three Screen Report* 7, no. 4 (2009): 2. http://in.nielsen.com/site/documents/3Screens_4Q09_US_rpt.pdf (accessed Feb. 13, 2011). / "What Consumers Watch: Nielsen's Q1 Three Screen Report." *Nielsenwire* (June 11, 2010). http://blog.nielsen.com/nielsenwire/online_mobile/what-consumers-watch-nielsens-q1-2010-three-screen-report/ (accessed Feb. 13, 2011).

2. Isra Deblauwe, "How Insectivorous are Gorillas?" *Gorilla Journal 33*, December 2006. http://www.berggorilla.de/english/gjournal/texte/33insect.html (accessed Feb. 13, 2011); D. Doran-Sheehy among others, "Male and Female Western Gorilla Diet: Preferred Foods, Use of Fallback Resources, and Implications for Ape Versus Old World Monkey Foraging Strategies." *Am J Phys Anthropol.* 140, no. 4 (December 2009): 727–38; I. Deblauwe and G.P. Janssens, "New Insights in Insect Prey Choice by Chimpanzees and Gorillas in Southeast Cameroon: The Role of Nutritional Value." *Am J Phys Anthropol.* 135, no. 1 (January 2008) : 42–55; A. Elgart-Berry, "Fracture Toughness of Mountain Gorilla (Gorilla gorilla beringei) Food Plants." *Am J Primatol.* 62, no. 4 (April 2004): 275–85; M.E. Rogers among others, "Western Gorilla Diet: A Synthesis from Six Sites." *Am J Primatol.* 64, no. 2

(October 2004): 173–92; J. Yamagiwa and A.K. Basabose, "Diet and Seasonal Changes in Sympatric Gorillas and Chimpanzees at Kahuzi-Biega National Park." *Primates.* 47, no. 1 (January 2006): 74–90. Epub 2005 Sep 3; D. Fossey and A.H. Harcourt, "Feeding Ecology of Free Ranging Mountain Gorillas (Gorilla gorilla beringei)" in Clutton Brock (ed.), *Primate Ecology: Studies of feeding and ranging behaviour in lemurs, monkeys and apes.* 1977. London: Academic Press; "Gorilla Conservation." *WAZA magazine.* World Association of Zoos and Aquariums. 11 (2009): 4, 23–4. http://www.yog2009.org/YoG_Downloads/WAZA_mag11_gorillas.pdf (accessed Feb. 13, 2011).

3.   M.A. Huffman, "Animal Self-medication and Ethno-medicine: Exploration and Exploitation of the Medicinal Properties of Plants." *Proc Nutr Soc.* 62, no. 2 (May 2003): 371–81.

4.   D.G. Popovich among others, "The Western Lowland Gorilla Diet has Implications for the Health of Humans and other Hominoids." *J Nutr.* 127, no. 19 (October 1997): 2000–5.

5.   "Secret of Long Life in Okinawa." CNN You Tube. http://www.youtube.com/watch?v=ZwX9Ll19cX0&feature=player_embedded (accessed Feb. 13, 2011).

6.   Sanjay Gupta, "Western Diet: A Killer in Okinawa. Part II." Vita+Signs, CNN You Tube. http://www.youtube.com/watch?v=8teAABsnTmM&feature=related (accessed Feb. 13, 2011).

7.   B. Strasser among others, "Efficacy of Systematic Endurance and Resistance Training on Muscle Strength and Endurance Performance in Elderly Adults – A Randomized Controlled Trial." *Wien Klin Wochenschr.* 121, no. 23-24 (2009): 757–64.

8.   Carmen Castaneda Sceppa and Jennifer Layne, "Low Protein + Low Exercise = Sarcopenia." *Agricultural Research Magazine.* 53, no. 5 (2005): 14–16. http://www.ars.usda.gov/is/AR/archive/may05/sarco0505.htm (accessed Feb. 13, 2011). http://www.ars.usda.gov/is/AR/archive/may05/sarco0505.pdf (accessed Feb. 13, 2011).

9.   J.D. Moreland among others, "Muscle Weakness and Falls in Older Adults: A Systematic Review and Meta-analysis." *J Am Geriatr Soc.* 52, no. 7 (July 2004): 1121–9; W.J. Evans, "What is Sarcopenia?" *J Gerontol A Biol Sci Med Sci.* 50, Spec No (November 1995): 5–8; P. Szulc among others, "Low Skeletal Muscle Mass is Associated with Poor Structural Parameters of Bone and Impaired Balance in Elderly Men – The MINOS Study." *J Bone Miner Res.* 20, no. 5 (May 2005): 721–9. Epub 2004 Dec 20; T. Lang among others, "Sarcopenia: Etiology, Clinical Consequences, Intervention, and Assessment." *Osteoporos Int.* 21, no. 4 (April 2010): 543–559.

10. Kirk Hamilton, "Aging, Sarcopenia (Muscle Loss) and Creatine Supplementation." Interview with Chad M. Kerksick, *Expert Speak* interviews

at Vitasearch.com. http://www.vitasearch.com/CP/experts/KerksickC-MAT2010-01-20.pdf (accessed Feb. 13, 2011).

11. W.J. Evans, "Reversing Sarcopenia: How Weight Training can Build Strength and Vitality." *Geriatrics*. 51, no. 5 (May 1996): 46-7, 51–3; quiz 54; M.A. Rogers and W.J. Evans, "Changes in Skeletal Muscle with Aging: Effects of Exercise Training." *Exerc Sport Sci Rev*. 21 (1993): 65–102; W.J. Evans and W.W. Campbell, "Sarcopenia and Age-related Changes in Body Composition and Functional Capacity." *J Nutr*. 123 (2 Suppl), (February 1993): 465–8.

12. W.J. Evans, "What is Sarcopenia?" *J Gerontol A Biol Sci Med Sci*. 50, Spec No (November 1995): 5–8.

13. Jennifer Cheeseman Day, "Population Projections of the United States, by Age, Sex, Race, and Hispanic Origin: 1993 to 2050." *Current Population Reports*, P25-1104, U.S. Bureau of the Census, U.S. Government Printing Office, 1993. http://www.census.gov/prod/1/pop/profile/95/24_ps.pdf (accessed Feb. 13, 2011). http://www.census.gov/population/www/pop-profile/elderpop.html (accessed Feb. 13, 2011); *Aging*. World Health Organization. http://www.who.int/topics/ageing/en/ (accessed Feb. 13, 2011).

14. The Nielsen Company, "What Consumers Watch: Americans Spend More Time with Video Than Ever Consumers devote 3.5 hours a month to using TV and the Internet simultaneously." *Three Screen Report* 7, no. 4 (2009): 2. http://in.nielsen.com/site/documents/3Screens_4Q09_US_rpt.pdf (accessed Feb. 13, 2011). / "What Consumers Watch: Nielsen's Q1 Three Screen Report." *Nielsenwire* (June 11, 2010). http://blog.nielsen.com/nielsenwire/online_mobile/what-consumers-watch-nielsens-q1-2010-three-screen-report/ (accessed Feb. 13, 2011).

Chapter 15
The TRIAD Mind-Body Program

1. Marc Allen, *The Greatest Secret of All: Moving Beyond Abundance to a Life of True Fulfillment*. (Novato, California: New World Library, 2008).

2. Jack Canfield, *The Success Principles: How to Get from Where You Are to Where You Want to Be*. First Collins paperback edition. (New York: HarperCollins, 2007), 23.

Appendix B
Anti-Inflammatory Diet Principles

1. Jens Kjeldsen-Kragh among others, "Controlled Trial of Fasting and One Year Vegetarian Diet in Rheumatoid Arthritis." *Lancet.* 338 (Oct. 12, 1991): 899–902; I. Hafstrom among others, "A Vegan Diet Free of Gluten Improves the Signs and Symptoms of Rheumatoid Arthritis: The Effects on Arthritis Correlate With a Reduction in Antibodies to Food Antigens." *Rheumatology.* 40 (2001): 1175–9.

2. Joel Fuhrman, B. Sarter, and D.J. Calabro, "Brief Case Reports of Medically Supervised, Water–Only Fasting Associated With Remission of Autoimmune Disease." *Alternative Therapies.* 8, no. 4 (Jul.–Aug. 2002): 112, 140, 111; O. Adam, "Anti-Inflammatory Diet and Rheumatic Diseases." *European Journal of Clinical Nutrition.* 49 (1995): 703–17; O. Adam among others, "Anti-Inflammatory Effects of a Low Arachidonic Acid Diet and Fish Oil in Patients With Rheumatoid Arthritis." *Rheumatology International.* 23 (2003): 27–36; I. Hafstrom among others, "A Vegan Diet Free of Gluten Improves the Signs and Symptoms of Rheumatoid Arthritis: The Effects on Arthritis Correlate With a Reduction in Antibodies to Food Antigens." *Rheumatology.* 40 (2001): 1175–9; Jens Kjeldsen-Kragh among others, "Controlled Trial of Fasting and One Year Vegetarian Diet in Rheumatoid Arthritis." *Lancet.* 338 (Oct. 12, 1991): 899–902; Chiaki Shigemitsu among others, "Effect of Vegetarian Diet on Systemic Lupus Erythematosus." *Lancet.* 339 (May 9, 1992): 1177.

3. Joel Fuhrman, B. Sarter, and D.J. Calabro, "Brief Case Reports of Medically Supervised, Water-Only Fasting Associated With Remission of Autoimmune Disease." *Alternative Therapies.* 8, no. 4 (Jul.–Aug. 2002): 112, 140, 111.

Index

Publisher's Contribution TO
INTERNATIONAL WATER & HEALTH ALLIANCES
(IWHA)

A portion of each
Staying Healthy in the Fast Lane
book sold will be donated to the
International Water & Health Alliances

IWHA is a nonprofit organization committed to disseminating information and tools, such as the *Portable Microbiology Laboratory*, to allow for community-administered water testing and solar and/or chemical water pasteurization efforts to be conducted worldwide to reduce water-borne disease, a needless and preventable cause of frequent hospitalizations and major healthcare expenditures in developing countries. The unique commitment of IWHA is giving the local community the power and knowledge to administer their own testing on demand, not only providing the ability to purify the water locally but also to learn what local environmental situations relate to their specific water sanitation issues.

It is *Prescription2000.com's* strong position that the prevention of water-borne disease by local community-driven detection and water pasteurization programs provided by the IWHA, along with education on the *Staying Healthy Today* principles demonstrated in the "*9 Simple Steps to Optimal Health*" of the **TRIAD Wellness Program**, will assist developing countries in providing the most cost-effective, efficient, prevention-oriented and sustainable healthcare to their people.

IWHA
P.O. BOX 332, DAVIS, CA 95616
INFO@WATERINTERNATIONAL.ORG